Ketogenic Diet Air Fryer Cookbook

Amazingly Quick, Easy And Delicious Low Carb Keto Diet Weight Loss Air Fried Recipes Made For Your Air Fryer Everyday Cooking

By Coco Clark

© Copyright 2018 -Coco Clark -All rights reserved.

In no way is it legal to reproduce, duplicate, or transmit any part of this document by either electronic means or in printed format. Recording of this publication is strictly prohibited, and any storage of this material is not allowed unless with written permission from the publisher. All rights reserved.

The information provided herein is stated to be truthful and consistent, in that any liability, regarding inattention or otherwise, by any usage or abuse of any policies, processes, or directions contained within is the solitary and complete responsibility of the recipient reader. Under no circumstances will any legal liability or blame be held against the publisher for any reparation, damages, or monetary loss due to the information herein, either directly or indirectly. Respective authors own all copyrights not held by the publisher.

Legal Notice:
This book is copyright protected. This is only for personal use. You cannot amend, distribute, sell, use, quote or paraphrase any part or the content within this book without the consent of the author or copyright owner. Legal action will be pursued if this is breached.

Disclaimer Notice:
Please note the information contained within this document is for educational and entertainment purposes only. Every attempt has been made to provide accurate, up to date and reliable, complete information. No warranties of any kind are expressed or implied. Readers acknowledge that the author is not engaging in the rendering of legal, financial, medical or professional advice.

By reading this document, the reader agrees that under no circumstances are we responsible for any losses, direct or indirect, which are incurred as a result of the use of information contained within this document, including, but not limited to, —errors, omissions, or inaccuracies.

Table of Contents

Introduction 9
Chapter 1: About the Ketogenic Diet 12
    What is the Ketogenic Diet? 12
    Benefits of Keto Diet 13
    Reduced Appetite 13
    Anti-Aging 13
    Increase HDL Cholesterol 13
    Eliminate Sugar Cravings 13
    Weight Loss 13
    Increase Energy 14
    Ketogenic Diet FAQ 14
    1. What is Ketosis? 14
    2. How Can I Tell If I'm in Ketosis? 14
    3. What Kinds of Vitamins and Supplements Should I Take? 15
    4. Will I Lose Muscle? 15
    5. Can I Eat Carbs Again? 15
    6. Can I Drink Alcohol? 15
    7. What Are Things That Can Disrupt Ketosis? 15
    8. I'm Not Losing Any Weight. What Do I Do? 16
    9. Is Exercise Necessary to Lose Weight? 16
    10. Can I Eat Fruit? 16
    11. Can I Build Muscle While in Ketosis? 16
    12. Can I Use Sweetener? 17
    13. How Many Carbs Should I Consume? 17
    Tips and Cautions for the Keto Diet 17

1. Stay Hydrated 17
2. Clean Your Pantry 17
3. Start Shopping 17
4. Make Sure You Take Salt 18
5. Decrease Stress 18
6. Plan Your Meals 18
7. Exercise 18
8. Don't Add Too Much Protein 18
Mistakes that Often Happen 19
Mistake 1: Not Being Ready for "Keto Flu" 19
Mistake 2: Not Exercising 20
Mistake 3: Trying to Shed Tons of Pounds in a Short Amount of Time 20
Mistake 4: Eating Too Much Junk, Processed, and Unhealthy Foods 20
Mistake 5: Insufficient Nutritional Needs 20
Foods to Eat and Avoid 21

Chapter 2: Everything About the Air Fryer 26
What is An Air Fryer? 26
The Benefits of The Air Fryers 27
Air Fryer vs. Traditional Fryer 28
The Various Air Fryer Brands 30
Phillips XL Air fryer 30
GoWISE USA GW22621 Electric Air Fryer 31
Power Air Fryer XL 31
Avalon Bay Digital Air Fryer 32
NuWave Brio Air Fryer 32
How to Use an Air Fryer 33
Preparation 33

Pre-Heating...33

Cooking..33

Cleaning...33

How to Clean & Maintain An Air Fryer..34

How to clean your air fryer...34

How to maintain your air fryer..34

How to Choose a Good Air Fryer...35

What affects the buyer's decision of your air fryer?...........................35

Tips on how to choose the air fryer best for you.................................36

Where to Buy a Good Air Fryer?..37

Air Frying Compatible Foods...37

Frozen Foods..37

Raw Meat...37

Vegetables...38

Baked Goods..38

Roasting Nuts..38

Wet-Battered Foods..38

FAQs of Air Fryer...38

1. Can we cook various kinds of food in the air fryer?.....................38

2. How long does it take to cook frozen foods?..................................39

3. How much can I cook in my air fryer?..39

4. Is there any specific kind of oils needed for air frying?.............39

5. Can I add more ingredients while the food is getting cooked in my air fryer?..39

6. Can I use a baking paper or aluminum foil in my air fryer?....39

7. Is preheating required before I cook?...39

Chapter 3: Air Fryer Breakfast Recipes..41

Delicious Breakfast Souffle...41

Yummy Breakfast Italian Frittata...42

Savory Cheese and Bacon Muffins..43

Best Air-Fried English Breakfast...44

Chapter 4: Air Fryer Lunch Recipes...45

Incredible Air-Fried Burgers..45

Extraordinary Stuffed Zucchini with Bacon and Jalapeno.................................. 46

Good-Tasting Turkey Rolls.. 47

Chapter 5: Air Fryer Dinner Recipes...48

General Wong's Beef and Broccoli..48

Irresistible Meatloaf..49

Rockstar Rib Eye-Steak... 50

Super-Yummy Roast Pork Belly...51

Outstanding Rack of Lamb.. 52

Phenomenal Herbed Roast Beef...53

Amazing Lamb Chops with Herbed Garlic Sauce... 54

Chapter 6: Air Fryer Appetizer Recipes...55

Astonishing Chicken Kebabs 55

Appetizing Avocado Fries 56

Godly Pork Taquitos... 57

Gratifying Stuffed Mushrooms...58

Everyday Chicken Nuggets.. 59

Chapter 7: Air Fryer Poultry Recipes.. 60

Flavorful Fried Chicken... 60

Delectable Whole Roast Chicken... 61

Divine Buffalo Wings.. 62

Flavorsome Honey Lime Chicken Wings.. 63

Delightful Coconut Crusted Chicken Tenders... 64

Well-Tasted Popcorn Chicken.. 65

Easy Chicken Strips... 66

Savory Sriracha Chicken Drumsticks... 67

Chinese-Style Honey Garlic Chicken.. 68

Rich Parmesan Crusted Chicken Breasts... 69

Nashville Flaming Hot Breaded Chicken.. 70

Desirable Korean Fried Chicken Wings.. 72

Awesome Crispy Baked Garlic Parmesan Chicken Wings....................................... 73

Spicy Teriyaki Chicken Wings.. 74

Chapter 8: Air Fryer Fish and Seafood... 75

Remarkable Fish and Chips with Sauce... 75

Grand Air-Fried Coconut Shrimp... 77

Splendid Salmon Patties... 78

Japanese-Style Fried Prawns... 79

Great Air-Fried Soft-Shell Crab.. 80

Stunning Air-Fried Clams... 81

Mind-Blowing Air-Fried Crawfish with Cajun Dipping Sauce................................. 82

Southern-Air-Fried Cat Fish... 83

Wondrous Creole Fried Shrimp with Sriracha Sauce.. 84

Chapter 9: Air Fryer Meat Recipes... 86

Sweet and Spicy Montreal Steak.. 86

Stunning Chicken Sandwich... 87

Hearty Hot Dogs... 88

Sweet and Sour Pork.. 89

Yummy Rodeo Sirloin Steaks with Coffee Rub.. 91

Chapter 10: Air Fryer Vegetable and Sides Recipes... 92

Supreme Air-Fried Tofu... 92

Not Your Average Zucchini Parmesan Chips..93

Outstanding Batter-Fried Scallions.. 94

Delectable French Green Beans with Shallots and Almonds................................95

Super-Healthy Air-Fried Green Tomatoes..96

Luscious Air-Fried Broccoli Crisps...97

Chapter 11: Air Fryer Desert Recipes..98

Toothsome Caramel Cheesecake.. 98

Conclusion...100

Introduction

Hi friend! This is Coco Clark. Firstly, I'd like to thank and congratulate you for reading this book: "*Ketogenic Diet Air Fryer Cookbook- Amazingly Quick, Easy And Delicious Low Carb Keto Diet Air Fried Recipes Made For Your Air Fryer Everyday Cooking*". I hope this book will bring you the support and guidance you're looking for!

Please allow me ask you some questions:

Are you tired from all of your failed weight loss attempts?

Do you find that exercising just doesn't seem to help?

Do you want to enjoy fried foods and still maintain yet a healthier version of your body?

Are you tired of wasting time and oil in the kitchen?

Are you searching for an easy-to-use kitchen gadget that can bake, grill, and fry in a matter of minutes?

If you answered yes to any of the above, then you are certainly at the right spot. Keep reading! You will find all the answers!

Just the thought of dieting, attempting weight loss, and getting healthy leaves most of us feeling unmotivated and daunted.

But the ketogenic diet is a proven, effective and natural diet that can help kickstart your weight loss and allow for steady progress over time. The keto diet and the Air Fryer are a perfect pairing that allows you to prepare quick, healthy, and delicious meals and achieve a much healthier lifestyle.

The ketogenic diet works on a simple principle: it causes your body to switch from its preferred fuel source, carbohydrates, to fat, by entering the metabolic state called "ketosis". When your body is in ketosis, it will quickly burn through the limited carbs you consume and will mostly rely on fat from your diet and from the fat stores in your body. In addition, ketogenic diets have been proven to help decrease appetite and cravings, elevate your blood sugar, help control your blood pressure, increase your lifespan, and speed up your metabolism.

This book contains proven steps and strategies on how to use your Air Fryer to make ketogenic recipes, faster than ever. These easy Air Fryer recipes are simple to make, taste delicious, and give a multitude of nutrients to keep you happy and healthy. According to common belief, using the Air Fryer requires an advanced set of cooking skills, but that's completely untrue! This book will teach you how to use it to prepare food faster. With your Air Fryer, you'll be eating healthy and keto-friendly foods every day without spending too much time in the kitchen. So, let's get started!

Chapter 1: About the Ketogenic Diet

The following chapter will cover everything you need to know about following the ketogenic diet. The ketogenic diet is not like any other diet; it's medically safe and can help make you lose a lot of weight and ultimately change your life. However, it's not a miracle diet. It's still going to take work and discipline.

In this chapter, you will learn everything you need to know about the diet itself.

What is the Ketogenic Diet?

The ketogenic diet is a diet that's very low in carbohydrates and very high in fats, which is designed to force the body to produce ketones as an alternative source of energy. Glucose is the primary source of fuel for the body, because it's the easiest to break down and convert into energy. When your body makes glucose, it also produces insulin to help process glucose and distribute it through your body through your blood sugar levels. The more insulin is produced, the more glucose in your bloodstream.

Since your body has been using carbs for energy, fat is stockpiled in the body. Fat storage is also prompted by your body's insulin output: more insulin, more fat stored. What the ketogenic diet does is deprive your body of carbohydrates so it has no other choice but to use fat as its new source of energy. The standard ketogenic diet has a low carbohydrate intake, high protein, and high fat. The composition of food intake would be 5% carbs, 20% protein, and 75% fat.

Benefits of Keto Diet

The ketogenic diet is proven to have medical and health benefits. The diet was originally pioneered in the 1900s as a way of treating diabetes; once insulin was discovered, it became the medicine of choice because it allowed diabetics to eat a "normal" diet; but the benefits of the ketogenic diet remain indisputable. The aim of this diet is to maintain the metabolic state of ketosis. While under ketosis, you are burning ketones for energy, rather than carbohydrates. This comes with numerous of benefits such as:

Reduced Appetite: One of the biggest benefits is that the ketogenic diet keeps you fuller for a longer period of time. The ketogenic diet consists of mainly protein and fats which helps you feel satiated.

Anti-Aging: Lowering your insulin levels can increase your lifespan and help you appear more youthful.

Increase HDL Cholesterol: The ketogenic diet will increase your "good" cholesterol. This will help in reducing the risk of heart disease. It also helps lower your blood pressure and sugar levels, which, in turn, help lower your risk of diabetes and kidney failures.

Eliminate Sugar Cravings: Another benefit is that you will lose your sugar cravings; you'll only feel hungry when your body actually needs food, so you can trust your hunger once more, and eat when hungry.

Weight Loss: The keto diet does this in two ways: it reduces your appetite and cravings, so by eating when hungry you will often naturally reduce your calorie intake. Also, ketosis causes your body to burn fat as fuel. The diet is also slightly diuretic (promotes urine production), so you will lose some water weight.

Increase Energy: The body is more efficient at burning fat rather than carbohydrates, providing an increase in energy. Many people report an increase in energy, positive mood and productivity once they're fully accustomed to the keto diet.

Ketogenic Diet FAQ

In this section, you will find answers to some of the most frequently asked questions. Here is a reference guide for every time something enters your mind.

1. What is Ketosis?
Ketosis is the metabolic state where your body adjusts to burning fat (ketones) for fuel rather than carbohydrates (glucose).

2. How Can I Tell If I'm in Ketosis?
You can test your ketone levels with urine strips, breath tests (on ketosis, your breath may smell like acetone), or blood tests. You can also go by the symptoms of decreased appetite, improved focus and more energy. While starting ketosis, you may experience side effects like fatigue; these should clear up within a few days as your body adjusts.

3. What Kinds of Vitamins and Supplements Should I Take?

People who are first starting the keto diet will go through numerous body changes. Before taking new supplements, always consult your doctor. The following supplements are worth considering, but not mandatory:

- Multivitamins
- Vitamin D supplement
- Vitamin B Complex
- Magnesium Supplement
- Potassium Supplement

4. Will I Lose Muscle?

Any diet comes with the risk of muscle loss; the keto diet is not riskier than other diets, and may even be less risky, since you will be increasing your protein intake. If you are worried, try lifting weights for exercise.

5. Can I Eat Carbs Again?

Yes, eventually you can increase your carb intake; however, you must eliminate carbs entirely when starting this diet. Give yourself 3 months before you slowly reintroduce carbs. You will still need to stay below 50g of carbs per day in order to stay on a low-carb diet.

6. Can I Drink Alcohol?

Yes, you can drink alcohol, but it may take longer to lose weight. Beer and wine should be avoided because of the sugar and carbs they contain; spirits are preferable. Even so, it's better to limit your alcohol intake.

7. What Are Things That Can Disrupt Ketosis?

There are many things that can put you out of ketosis, such as consumption of sugar, soda, grains and other carbs. Starchy vegetables, lack of physical activity, artificial sweeteners, and too much protein can also be damaging for ketosis as well. Fortunately, the body can recover quickly; ketosis can resume within a day or so, so if you fall off the wagon, don't worry. Just try to return to your health eating!

8. I'm Not Losing Any Weight. What Do I Do?

This is very common for some practitioners. Here are some things that you should consider:

- Keep track of your macronutrient ratios. Make sure you are getting your energy requirements daily.
- Follow a keto diet plan; no snacking or extra carbs.
- Make sure you are adding physical activity to your lifestyle.
- Try intermittent fasting.

9. Is Exercise Necessary to Lose Weight?

Not necessarily; however, exercise will help immensely. While under ketosis, you will shed pounds quickly as a matter of course, but exercise is good for building muscle tone and overall health. Try moderate cardio such as walking or light cycling and strength training to build muscle.

10. Can I Eat Fruit?

Yes, you can eat some fruits, such as avocados, coconut and limited amounts of berries. However, most fruits contain too much sugar.

11. Can I Build Muscle While in Ketosis?

Yes, you can build muscle, but it will be harder and you may need a bodybuilding program designed specifically for keto dieters. The keto diet generally does not support high-intensity cardio workouts (which generally requires a steady glucose supply) and it can be more difficult to build muscle, so bodybuilders may choose to "carb-load" on workout days, in order to support their goals.

12. Can I Use Sweetener?
You can use sweetener. However, use natural low-carb sweeteners such as stevia and erythritol.

13. How Many Carbs Should I Consume?
Your diet must consist of no more than 5-10% of carbohydrates. So, on average, aim for 15-30 grams of net carbs per day.

Tips and Cautions for the Keto Diet

Your main goal on the ketogenic diet is to maintain the state of ketosis. However, this may be more challenging to some. Here are some of the best tips for following the ketogenic diet and maintaining ketosis:

1.Stay Hydrated: Staying hydrated by drinking a lot of water is essential for any diet. Water flushes the toxins out of your body, keeps your energy levels up, and keeps you in a good mood. Make sure that you are at least drinking eight 8-ounce glasses of water per day.

2.Clean Your Pantry: Get rid of the old so that you can bring the new food in. It's not going to help you if you have unhealthy foods tempting you each time you enter the kitchen. Get rid of all the starches and grains such as cereal, pasta, rice, flour, bread, etc. Get rid of sugary foods, soda, milk, fruit juices, candy, desserts and anything else.

3.Start Shopping: Restock your kitchen. Stock lots of meat such as pork, turkey, beef, lamb, chicken, and also eggs. Always keep a supply of non-starchy vegetables such as mushrooms, cucumbers, broccoli, asparagus, lettuce, peppers, tomatoes, onions, garlic, and cauliflower. Buy healthy fats and oils such as all-natural butter, avocado oil, coconut oil, or olive oil.

4. Make Sure You Take Salt: Salt is essential. Make sure you consume at least 2 teaspoons of salt per day. You can do this by drinking a cup of bouillon (hot water with a stock cube dissolved in it) or even just salt water. Don't hold back on seasoning your meals with salt, but also make sure you're not overdoing it. I recommend Himalayan salt as it has additional minerals and nutrients, and tastes great.

5. Decrease Stress: Stress is extremely damaging to your health. Stress can make it difficult to lose weight and can even lead you to gain weight. Try meditating, yoga, and deep breathing. These things can help eliminate stress and make the keto diet much easier.

6. Plan Your Meals: It's good to know when you're going to eat, what you're going to eat and even to do meal prep ahead of time. Having a meal plan provides a sense of direction on where to head with your diet, making it less intimidating. There are also recipes in this book that can be substituted for others in your meal plan. But do remember that caloric goals don't need to be precise. The keto diet does not encourage calorie counting.

7. Exercise: You will still need to add exercise to your ketogenic diet if you want to lose weight. If you don't exercise, your weight loss will be slower. Adopt a regular exercise regime – whatever activities you like the best - that combines both strength-training exercises and cardio exercises to maintain ketosis.

8. Don't Add Too Much Protein: Protein must make up no more than 30% of your calorie consumption. If you eat too much protein, your body will transform the amino acids into glucose through a process known as gluconeogenesis. Keep track of your macronutrients to help avoid eating too much protein.

Mistakes that Often Happen

The keto diet can be tough to get used to, and there are plenty of mistakes that you can make while you're on it. However, the keto diet is perfectly safe and healthy if you're doing it right. Here are the most common mistakes that starters often make and how you can avoid them.

Mistake 1: Not Being Ready for "Keto Flu"

The most challenging thing about starting the ketogenic diet is the keto flu, which refers to the side effects that you will experience while entering ketosis. The symptoms are flu-like, meaning fatigue and muscle aches, as well as brain fog, nausea, and lethargy.

As your body heads for ketosis, your body will undergo tons of changes. The most prominent is where your body starts to eliminate any stored sugars through urination. Frequent urination will lead to dehydration in many cases and when you urinate too frequently, you begin to release electrolytes. Thus, the keto flu can occur.

To avoid the keto flu, there are several things you can do:

- Drink plenty of soups and broths as these can bring back your electrolyte levels.
- Stir a teaspoon of salt into a glass of water, or season your meals with an extra teaspoon when cooking.
- Make sure you are getting enough magnesium by eating plenty of leafy greens.

- And finally, drink tons of water! Water is crucial for keeping your body running and staying well hydrated.

Mistake 2: Not Exercising

While reducing your calorie intake and allowing your body to burn fat instead of carbs is helping you lose weight, it's not the only factor. You need to keep active! Losing weight does not mean you are in shape! Exercising will make you stronger and increase the amount of work your heart can do, as well make you feel better as a whole. Find a workout regime you enjoy and stick with it!

Mistake 3: Trying to Shed Tons of Pounds in a Short Amount of Time

It is extremely unhealthy and even harmful to lose a lot of weight very quickly. Your body wasn't made for drastic change, and it can negatively affect your general wellness and cause you to lose muscle mass.

Not only is this extremely unhealthy, but it will leave you with loose skin and you will not be in proper shape. Be patient and treat yourself right. There's no need to rush; let the keto diet do its work.

Mistake 4: Eating Too Much Junk, Processed, and Unhealthy Foods

It's easy to be lazy and eat whatever is nearby. However, if you eat too much unhealthy food, you will find yourself exceeding your sodium intake. This can lead to higher blood pressure. Make sure you carefully monitor your sodium levels and limit your intake of junk, processed, and any non-keto foods.

Mistake 5: Insufficient Nutritional Needs

You need to make sure your body is taking in its proper vitamins and minerals. To ensure you do this, eat plenty of vegetables and leafy greens. Leafy greens are packed with dietary fiber which will help keep your body full for a longer period of time. You can also try using vitamin pills and supplements to take of your nutritional needs.

Foods to Eat and Avoid

In this chapter, you will learn what to eat and what not to eat. First, here is everything you are allowed to eat when following this diet:

Vegetables: You can eat all vegetables. Especially leafy green vegetables such as cabbage, lettuce, kale, and spinach. However, do your best to avoid eating potatoes, sweet potatoes, carrots, and parsnips as they are high in carbs. Other vegetables you can eat include:

- Artichoke Hearts
- Asparagus
- Avocados (extremely filling and full of fat)
- Broccoli
- Brussel Sprouts
- Cauliflower
- Celery
- Mushrooms (very low in carbs)
- Onions
- Peppers
- Zucchini
- Jalapenos
- Tomatoes

Meat, Fish, and Seafood: Meat is extremely important for the keto diet. Meat is full of protein and fat and consists of zero carbs, which means you can eat as much as you like. You can eat all meat which includes:

- Chicken
- Beef
- Pork
- Fish
- Lobster
- Shrimp
- Organ meats
- Chorizo (spicy sausage)
- Sardines
- Mackerel

Fats: Fats must take up most of your diet. You can find fats in coconut oil, olive oil, duck fat, butter, sesame oil, and ghee. You can also get your fats from oily fish, oils, meats, eggs, and avocados.

Nuts and Seeds: You are allowed to eat nuts and seeds but only in moderation. This includes:

- Pecans
- Walnuts
- Macadamia nuts
- Pine nuts
- Pumpkin seeds
- Sunflower seeds
- Flaxseeds
- Note: AVOID peanuts; they are a legume, not a nut.

Nuts can make you exceed the limit of your carbohydrate consumption, so limit your intake, and avoid salted nuts which are easy to overeat. You can also eat small quantities of dark chocolate and beef jerky.

Drinks: You can drink non-dairy milk such as coconut milk, almond milk, and cashew milk. You can also drink broth, stock, coffee without any sugar, herbal teas, and water.

Dairy: You are allowed to eat some dairy, but be extra attentive with your choices. If you want dairy in your diet, always go for full-fat choices such as cream yogurt, butter, and cheese. You should avoid milk because of its high lactose content.

Seasonings: You can use all seasonings, spices, and herbs.

When beginning your keto journey make sure you keep track of your carb intake. It is very easy to go above your carb limit with just a single meal!

Here are all the foods that you should avoid:

All Grains: Avoid all kinds of grains. This includes:

- Wheat
- Oats
- Corn
- Barley
- Rice
- Quinoa
- Potatoes
- Sugar
- Cakes

- Beer
- Pasta
- Bread
- Pizza
- Cookies
- Crackers

Avoid processed foods: Almost everything that comes in a box and wrapper. Always pick natural and whole foods if you can.

Avoid Refined Fats and Oils: This includes:

- Sunflower oil
- Canola oil
- Grapeseed oil
- Vegetable Oils
- Margarine

Avoid beans and legumes: This includes:

- Lentils
- Chickpeas
- Beans
- Green beans (you can eat in small quantities)
- Peas (you can eat in small quantities)

Avoid sugary drinks like soda, milkshakes, fruit juice, and cider.

Fruits: Avoid all kinds of fruits as they consist of too much sugar which is bad for maintaining ketosis. You are allowed to eat small quantities of blueberries, blackberries, gooseberries, raspberries, and strawberries.

Alcohol: You don't have to completely cut out alcohol, but things may get complicated if you are a frequent drinker, as it could lead to weight gain or delay weight loss. When you drink alcohol, your body processes the alcohol before anything else, so your body will put a halt on burning fat and process the alcohol instead. If you do want to enjoy alcohol, go for liquor without any added sugar or syrups. You can find these in whiskey, spiced rum, and tequila. If you want to enjoy beer, go for light beers or a brand with a low carb content.

Avoid salad dressings. If you can't eat a salad without a dressing, go for a homemade salad dressing that is keto friendly, or use olive oil or a vinegar dressing. Blue cheese dressing is low in carbs so it's a good choice.

Avoid commercial cheese spreads, coffee creamers, artificial sweeteners, condensed milk, soy milk, rice milk, syrups, sugar, and dried fruit.

There are plenty of things that you should avoid on the keto diet, but there are also tons of things you can eat. Always focus on the foods you can eat rather than the things you cannot.

Chapter 2: Everything About the Air Fryer

The air fryer is a modern kitchen gadget that uses the rapid circulation of hot air to cook foods through. If you are looking for healthy meals that are rich in texture, packed with flavor, nutrients, and low in fat, then using an air fryer would be the best choice. In this chapter, you will get to learn everything you need to know about air frying and how to use it as a professional.

What is An Air Fryer?

An air fryer is a one-of-a-kind conventional form of oven, almost the same size as a rice cooker. Cooking with an air fryer utilizes the rapid circulation of hot air around your meals (as the picture shows below). The circulation of heat moves at an incredibly high speed that it cooks quickly providing a crispy texture on the outside and a soft one the inside. Air fryers can fry, bake, roast, and grill any sorts of foods with the requirement of little to no oil at all.

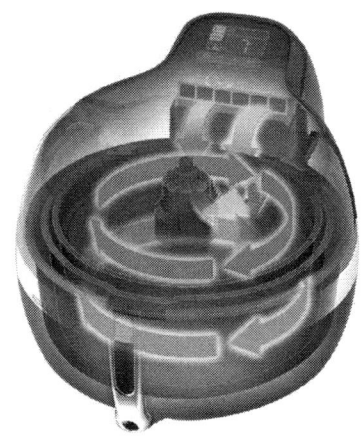

Also, the air fryers have a timer and an adjustable temperature manager which means that you do not need to keep a tab on your food as everything is done automatically. Using an air fryer is a matter of adding the meal, adjusting the temperature, and setting the time. Although some recipes may require a little extra care, other than that, it's most often a times a pretty much smooth sailing experience whenever it comes to using the air fryers.

The Benefits of The Air Fryers

There is an endless list of benefits when it comes to air frying, and below are some of them:

1. Air fryers can provide you with delicious and tasty meals every day at any time.

2. Air fryers avoid dry fried foods (common in deep fryers), while at the same time retains the crispy texture on the outside.

3. Air fryers can cook and heat foods in a matter of minutes.

4. Air fryers is multiple purpose kitchen device as it can fry, grill, roast, bake, and even make soups.

5. Air fryers are user-friendly appliance that comes with a timer, which means that you can cook your food and walk away without any fear of oil splattering or spillages, grease fires, burning, or foods sticking.

6. Air fryers saves money as you will be using lesser oil to fry foods.

7. Air fryers are low-maintenance and easily cleaned devices as most parts can be stripped and dish washed.

8. Air fryers can prepare foods with eighty percent less fat than oil fried foods, thus making it much healthier.

9. Air fryers contains a lid for frying which makes it one of the safest devices that everyone could use in frying.

Air Fryer vs. Traditional Fryer

The major discrepancies between the traditional and air fryers include:

The Oil Factor: With an air fryer, it requires little to no oil, or in rare cases only a tablespoon or two at most cases, while on the other hand, deep fryers need a lot of oil. A deep fryer typically requires 1 to 4 quarts of cooking oil which also requires a constant oil replacement at certain intervals, meaning that you will spending more money on oil.

The Health Factor: With an air fryer, you will be using an unnoticeable percentage of oil, thus making it much healthier by reducing the fat content to 80 percent other than in the case of using a deep fryer.

The Neatness Factor: Air fryers have a dishwasher safe removable cooking component and is also easy to clean up. All that is required with an air fryer is to clean the cooking basket, cooking pan, and the drip pan which can all easily done by hand.

But in the case of using the deep fryers, oil vapors can settle on the counter top, kitchen walls, and even the floors, making it messy and detrimental to ones health. Thus, you will spend more time cleaning these surfaces. Also, cleaning the deep fryer is not easy, depending on the brand, some parts may or may not be safe to dish wash, and some areas may be impossible to reach.

The Safety Factor: Air frying is safe to use, because your cooking will be done while the food is covered with a lid. It can prepare foods without the need for you to stand beside it. However, when using a deep fryer, you need to stand in front of the hot oil to cook. Using the deep fryer carries more risk as the oil can splatter making the floors slippery, flickering on your skin, and even grease fire. Foods can also get burnt in the hot oil whereas with an air fryer you will just need to set the temperature, timer and walk away.

The Versatility Factor: Air fryers have multiple uses compared to the deep fryers. You can fry, grill, roast, and bake in your air fryers whereas you can use only deep fries in a deep fryer.

The Taste Factor: Deep fryers have a crunchier texture compared to the air fryers, because deep fryers are suitable for wet battered foods. In an air fryer, using wet batter foods will make the batter splatter, implying that to obtain a more crunchier texture, you will need to add an additional tablespoon of oil to your meals using an air fryer. The only difference would be the degree of crunchiness of the skin and of course the fat content.

The Time Factor: Deep frying is quicker than air frying. With deep fryers, heat is rapidly transferred from the hot oil to the food items. French fries will take around 10 to 15 minutes in your air fryer but only a couple of minutes in your deep fryer.

The Capacity Factor: Deep fryers generally have a large capacity than air fryers. If you are the type that cooks in large quantities (6+ servings), then deep fryers should be your most preferable. Air fryers is suitable for 2 to 4 servings at most.

The Reheating Factor: You can reheat foods in your air fryer in a matter of minutes compared to deep fryers. With deep fryers, it would not be so practical, because you will need to undergo the process of preparing the oil and cleaning afterward for just a small portion of food. Air fryers are more convenient and practical for reheating.

The Cost Factor: Air fryers are more costly than the deep fryers ranging from $50 to under $200 for the more expensive models. The air fryers cost more with most of the brands ranging from $100 to $200.

The Various Air Fryer Brands

Here is a list of some air fryer brands in the market. Find out which one is the best for you:

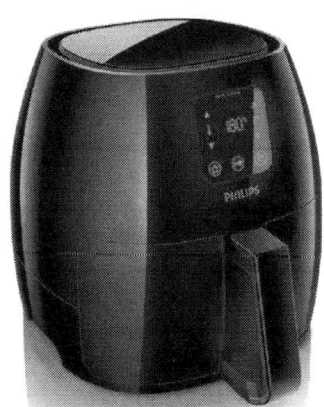

Phillips XL Air fryer: This air fryer has a large capacity making it a perfect choice for families or anyone who wishes to fry huge batches at once. This air fryer brand is also good for roasting, baking, and steaming ingredients. It comes with a dishwasher-safe for a smooth clean-up, a touch-screen interface, an adjustable temperature up to 390 degrees, and a 60-minute timer.

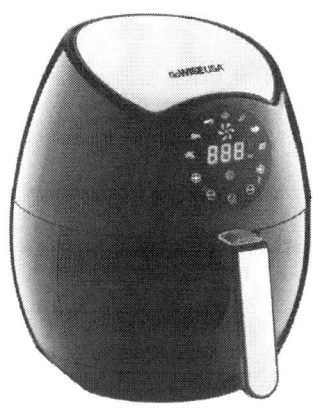

GoWISE USA GW22621 Electric Air Fryer: This brand has an adjustable temperature range of 175 to 390 degrees and can cook meals under 30 minutes. This air fryer is a practical choice for smaller families or for anyone who doesn't cook large batches frequently. The touchscreen is simple and has seven inbuilt programs. You can pick from the general food items including chips, chicken, fish, fries, and meat.

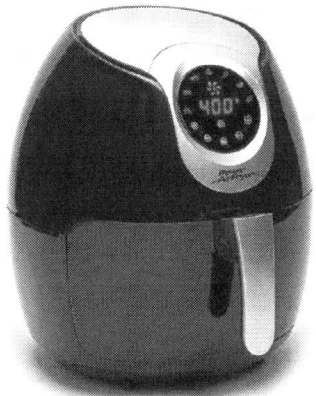

Power Air Fryer XL: This air fryer uses cyclonic heated air which cooks foods precisely and evenly for a delicious savory result without using any added oil. Other than that it comprises of an automated touch screen, and seven presets for popular meal items including chicken, fries, steaks, and baking goods.

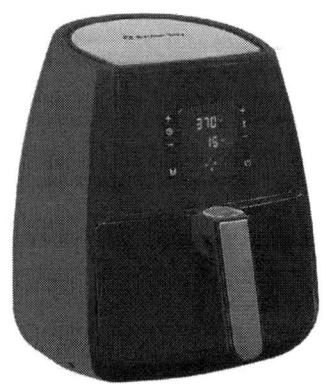

Avalon Bay Digital Air Fryer: This brand comes with a fan that removes excess fats and oils from the food before air frying. The circulated air is then moved at a high speed to cook and heat the food efficiently for an even result. Also, this air fryer is perfect for baking, roasting, and grilling food items. The temperature for this brand ranges from 200 to 400 degrees and some customers claim you can use wet-battered ingredients with no expected splattering effects. It also has a non-slip rubber pad to hold the air fryer firmly in place.

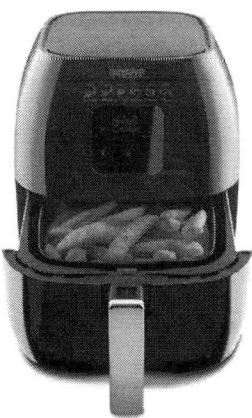

NuWave Brio Air Fryer: This air fryer is good for cooking foods faster and simpler. This brand comes with of a preheat function, which brings the fryer to the best possible cooking temperature for your foods. It also has a digital touch screen to adjust the temperature and time.

Also in this brand to ensure safety, the air frying process won't begin until the fry bucket is fully locked.

How to Use an Air Fryer

There are 4 steps in using an air fryer, follow this set of instructions when cooking anything with it:

Preparation: To prevent ingredients from sticking to the air fryer basket, spray it with a nonstick cooking spray or add a tablespoon of oil. Don't over pack foods in your air fryer basket otherwise some parts won't be fully cooked thoroughly. If you are working with a marinated or wet ingredients, make sure you rub them dry, because this will help avert splattering or excess smoke.

Pre-Heating: Plug in your air fryer and preheat it. This usually takes around five minutes, although preheating is not that necessary, nevertheless it can reduce your time in cooking.

Cooking: If you are cooking frozen foods or items with small ingredients, try shaking the air fryer many times to prepare it evenly and efficiently. Also when cooking high fatty foods, you should have it at the back of your mind that, the fats will drop to the base of the air fryer, which will thereafter need cleaning.

Cleaning: To ensure your air fryer stays in shape, make sure you clean it properly by purifying the air fryer basket and the pan after using them. Most air fryers come with dishwasher safe parts which makes this process easy.

How to Clean & Maintain An Air Fryer

The first thing you should have at your finger tips is that, if you do not clean and maintain your air fryer from time to time, it won't last long. Following these guidelines will secure the fact that your air fryer will remain effective and durable for years to come.

How to clean your air fryer

Unplug your air fryer from the wall socket and allow it to cool until you can touch.

Using a wet rag, wipe the exterior part of your air fryer.

Remove the air fryer pan, tray, basket and wash it with hot water and a dishwasher soap in your sink. These parts are removable and are safe for an easy cleanup.

Use a cloth or sponge to wipe and clean the inner part of your air fryer.

If you find any ingredients sticking in your air fryer, scrub it off with a brush.

Before adding the pan, tray, and basket back into your air fryer ensure they are entirely dry.

Once your air fryer is cleaned, store it safely.

How to maintain your air fryer

Your air fryer requires a standard form of maintenance to ensure it does not get damaged or work erroneously. To do this, one needs to follow this instructions:

Before using your air fryer, make sure you check the cord. That is, do not plug a damaged cord into an outlet; this can result in a ghastly injury or even death.

Make sure your air fryer is clean and free of any debris before you begin cooking. Check the inner part and make sure you remove anything redundant in there.

Ensure the air fryer is placed upright, on a flat surface.

Make sure that your air fryer is not too close to the wall or another appliance. Air fryers require 4-inches of space all around them.

One after the other, check each component of your air fryer, including the basket, pan, and handle.

If you find anything damaged or wrong with your air fryer, reach the manufacturer and get it replaced.

How to Choose a Good Air Fryer

There are wide varieties of air fryers available to you. The smartest choice will be to purchase from popular brands like Phillips, Kalorik, or some special air fryer brands recommended by experts and professionals. Here is some more insight when it comes to ordering your air fryer.

What affects the buyer's decision of your air fryer?

The increasing revenue of air fryers has reaped from its benefits of making healthy and low-cholesterol meals. With this you can cook fried chicken and potato chips that are healthy, nutritious, and less toxic than those of traditionally fried foods. Other benefits of air frying include fast cooking and an easy to use interface that it presents in your kitchen. With all this, who wouldn't buy an air fryer?

Tips on how to choose the air fryer best for you.

When it comes to owning an air fryer, there are some things you should have in in mind:

The size of your air fryer: The perfect sized air fryer gives your kitchen an enough space to serve, cook, and eat. To figure out the right size, you should have in mind that the ordinary air fryer can accommodate around 1.5 to 2 pounds of food items.

The capacity of your air fryer: Air fryers are electrically operated. Hence, inconsistencies in wattage stock can spark damage and electric shocks in your kitchen. Most standard ranges of air fryer capacity are from 700 to 1500 watts.

Controlling and signaling points: A good air fryer should have a digital touchscreen interface that can adjust temperature and time as well as switch modes. A timer is required to ensure fast and safe cooking. Some additional features should be checked for as it is going to give more comfort throughout your day to day cooking.

Warranty: Like any other device, buying gadgets will be more valuable due to its concentrated and considerate warranty terms. Having a warranty on your air fryer will be better than buying an air fryer without one. It is also preferable to purchase air fryers with full package home delivery.

The cost of your air fryer: Though an air fryer is highly recommended, it is costly compared to other kitchen gadgets. This is because of its level of utility as it prevents any form of grease fires, burns, and injury. The cost of air fryers is the most challenging factor for many and as such it is advisable that you should choose types that will lie within the whims and caprices of your budget.

It is also important to know that no matter the brand or price, all air fryers perform the same task irrespective. They all follow the principle of circulating hot air to cook and heat foods together. And so, your choice of an air fryer should not depend on technology or functions, but on the points mentioned above. Quality air fryers last longer and serve your needs better than investing in a cheaper module.

Where to Buy a Good Air Fryer?

There are many ways you can purchase an air fryer. Once you decide on the brand, you can Google and search up their websites. Alternatively, you can purchase air fryers on Amazon, online stores, and even grocery stores in their kitchen appliances section.

Air Frying Compatible Foods

Here is a list of compatible Air Frying foods:

Frozen Foods: Any kind of frozen foodstuff intended for baking purposes is a perfect fit for the air fryer. frozen things like fries, nuggets, and fish sticks cooks faster in your air fryer compared to your oven. And since there is no oil involved, it will lead to a low calories meal. For instance, French fries take around 12 minutes to achieve the crispy texture on the outside and a soft texture on the inside. You can shake the foods halfway through to ensure proper cooking and browning.

Raw Meat: You can roast any sort of meat in your air fryer, whether chicken, steak, pork, lamb, etc. A whole chicken will typically take about half an hour at 360 degrees F. to get done.

Vegetables: You can cook almost all forms of vegetables in your air fryer. Vegetables that you would normally grill can be done in your air fryer, and these includes cauliflower, green beans, onions, bell peppers can be all grilled in your air fryer.

Baked Goods: You can buy a nonstick baking dish along with your air fryer which is very useful when it comes to baking muffins, bread, lasagna, quiche, small cakes, or any other baked goods. This means you can bake anything you usually do in your oven using your air fryer with a more quicker and effective experience.

Roasting Nuts: Roasting nuts such as peanuts, walnuts, almonds, or any other kind of nuts can be easily done in your air fryer. This process will only take about 5 to 8 minutes, without it getting burned.

Wet-Battered Foods: Wet battered food is not suitable for air frying. The reason behind this is because the fast-moving air will burst the batter away from the food, causing it to splatter all over the cook basket,and creating a huge mess.

FAQs of Air Fryer

1. Can we cook various kinds of food in the air fryer?
Yes, you can easily prepare and cook any variety of foods in your air fryer. You can easily cook meats, potatoes, poultry, onion rings, and chicken nuggets .Aside from these things you can also bake cupcakes and grill vegetables.

2. How long does it take to cook frozen foods?
One of the great things about air frying frozen food is that it allows you to use the handle. But it usually takes more time to cook frozen foods compared to fresh ingredients.

3. How much can I cook in my air fryer?
This answer depends on the capacity of your air fryer. The majority of air fryers can hold up to 500 grams of food items. You can also see the max line of the basket on the air fryer which implies that the air fryer can be loaded up to that line.

4. Is there any specific kind of oils needed for air frying?
No, you don't need any special kind of oil for air frying. At most some recipes require a tablespoon or two of oil, of which you can use olive oil, coconut oil, vegetable oil, or butter spray.

5. Can I add more ingredients while the food is getting cooked in my air fryer?
Yes, you can add more ingredients while the food is getting cooked in your air fryer. However, be sure that the ingredients are added in the right away or else you may lose the heat which will result in an increase in the to cooking time.

6. Can I use a baking paper or aluminum foil in my air fryer?
Yes, you can use baking paper or aluminum foil, but you need to allocate some breathing space so that the steam can flow smoothly.

7. Is preheating required before I cook?
No, there is no need to preheat your air fryer. However, if you decide to preheat, it will take around 3 to 4 minutes and can help reduce the cooking time.

Now that we have known everything about the air fryer, let's cook some tasty and easy-to-make meals. It's effortless, all you have to do is just to follow the instructions properly. Also, do keep in mind that you are free to adjust the the recipes to your liking.

Chapter 3: Air Fryer Breakfast Recipes

Delicious Breakfast Souffle

Time: 20 minutes

Yield: 4

Ingredients:

- 6 eggs
- 1/3 of cup of milk
- ½ cup of shredded mozzarella cheese
- 1 tablespoon of freshly chopped parsley
- ½ cup of chopped ham
- 1 teaspoon of salt
- 1 teaspoon of black pepper
- ½ teaspoon of garlic powder

Instructions:

1. Grease 4 ramekins with a nonstick cooking spray.
2. Preheat your air fryer to 350 degrees Fahrenheit.
3. Using a large bowl, add and stir all the ingredients until it mixes properly.
4. Pour the egg mixture into the greased ramekins and place it inside your air fryer.
5. Cook it inside your air fryer for 8 minutes.
6. Then carefully remove the souffle from your air fryer and allow it to cool off.
7. Serve and enjoy!

Nutritional Information per serving:

Calories: 195, Fat: 15g, Protein: 9g, Carbohydrates: 6g, Dietary Fiber: 0.1g

Yummy Breakfast Italian Frittata

Time: 15 minutes

Yield: 4

Ingredients:

- 6 eggs
- 1/3 cup of milk
- 4-ounces of chopped Italian sausage
- 3 cups of stemmed and roughly chopped kale
- 1 red deseeded and chopped bell pepper
- ½ cup of a grated feta cheese
- 1 chopped zucchini
- 1 tablespoon of freshly chopped basil
- 1 teaspoon of garlic powder
- 1 teaspoon of onion powder
- 1 teaspoon of salt
- 1 teaspoon of black pepper

Instructions:

1. Preheat your air fryer to 360 degrees Fahrenheit.
2. Grease the air fryer pan with a nonstick cooking spray.
3. Add the Italian sausage to the pan and cook it inside your air fryer for 5 minutes.
4. While doing that, add and stir in the remaining ingredients until it mixes properly.
5. Add the egg mixture to the pan and allow it to cook inside your air fryer for 5 minutes.
6. Thereafter carefully remove the pan and allow it to cool off until it gets chill enough to serve.
7. Serve and enjoy!

Nutritional Information per serving:

Calories: 225, Fat: 14g, Protein: 20g, Dietary Fiber: 0.8g, Carbohydrates: 4.5g

Savory Cheese and Bacon Muffins

Time: 22 minutes

Yield: 4

Ingredients:

- 1 ½ cup of all-purpose flour
- 2 teaspoons of baking powder
- ½ cup of milk
- 2 eggs
- 1 tablespoon of freshly chopped parsley
- 4 cooked and chopped bacon slices
- 1 thinly chopped onion
- ½ cup of shredded cheddar cheese
- ½ teaspoon of onion powder
- 1 teaspoon of salt
- 1 teaspoon of black pepper

Instructions:

1. Preheat your air fryer to 360 degrees Fahrenheit.
2. Using a large bowl, add and stir all the ingredients until it mixes properly.
3. Then grease the muffin cups with a nonstick cooking spray or line it with a parchment paper. Pour the batter proportionally into each muffin cup.
4. Place it inside your air fryer and bake it for 15 minutes.
5. Thereafter, carefully remove it from your air fryer and allow it to chill.
6. Serve and enjoy!

Nutritional Information per serving:

Calories: 180, Fat: 18g, Protein: 15g, Dietary Fiber: 0.7g, Carbohydrates: 16g

Best Air-Fried English Breakfast

Time: 25 minutes

Yield: 4

Ingredients:

- 8 sausages
- 8 bacon slices
- 4 eggs
- 1 (16-ounce) can of baked beans
- 8 slices of toast

Instructions:

1. Add the sausages and bacon slices to your air fryer and cook them for 10 minutes at a 320 degrees Fahrenheit.
2. Using a ramekin or heat-safe bowl, add the baked beans, then place another ramekin and add the eggs and whisk.
3. Increase the temperature to 290 degrees Fahrenheit.
4. Place it inside your air fryer and cook it for an additional 10 minutes or until everything is done.
5. Serve and enjoy!

Nutritional Information per serving:

Calories: 850, Fat: 40g, Protein: 48g, Dietary Fiber: 18g,

Carbohydrates: 20g

Chapter 4: Air Fryer Lunch Recipes

Incredible Air-Fried Burgers

Time: 45 minutes

Yield: 4

Ingredients:

- 1 pound of lean ground beef
- 1 teaspoon of salt
- 1 teaspoon of black pepper
- 1 teaspoon of onion powder
- 1 teaspoon of garlic powder
- 1 tablespoon of freshly chopped or dried parsley
- 1 tablespoon of Worcestershire sauce

Instructions:

1. Preheat your air fryer to 390 degrees Fahrenheit.
2. Using a large bowl, add and mix all the ingredients until it is properly mixed.
3. Grease your air fryer cooking tray with a nonstick cooking spray.
4. Segment the ground beef mixture into four medium-sized patties and place it in the tray.
5. Place the tray inside your air fryer and cook it for 25 minutes.
6. After 25 minutes, flip the burgers and cook it for an additional 20 minutes.
7. Then gather your burgers and add any toppings you like.
8. Serve and enjoy!

Nutritional Information per serving:

Calories: 148, Fat: 5g, Protein: 24g, Dietary Fiber: 0.3g,

Carbohydrates: 1.7g

Extraordinary Stuffed Zucchini with Bacon and Jalapeno

Time: 15 minutes

Yield: 2

Ingredients:

- 3 zucchinis
- 6 cooked and crumbled bacon slices
- 1 chopped jalapeno
- 2 chopped tomatoes
- 1 (8-ounce) can of tomato sauce
- 1 cup of shredded mozzarella cheese
- 1 tablespoon of freshly chopped parsley
- 1 teaspoon of salt
- 1 teaspoon of black pepper

Instructions:

1. Cut the zucchini vertically and scoop out the inner portions.
2. Using a large bowl, add and mix the bacon, jalapeno, salt, black pepper, the parsley properly.
3. Pour in the tomatoes, the tomato sauce and stir until it mixes properly.
4. Fill the zucchini with the ground beef mixture and sprinkle it with the cheese
5. Place the stuffed zucchini in your air fryer basket and cook it for 10 minutes.
6. Serve and enjoy!

Nutritional Information per serving:

Calories: 210, Fat: 8g, Protein: 23g, Dietary Fiber: 2g,

Carbohydrates: 6g

Good-Tasting Turkey Rolls

Time: 40 minutes

Yield: 4

Ingredients:

- 2 tortilla wraps
- 2 cups of shredded leftover turkey breast
- 2 eggs
- 1 tablespoon of honey
- 1 tablespoon of soy sauce
- 1 tablespoon of Chinese five-spice
- 1 teaspoon of Worcester sauce
- 1 teaspoon of salt
- 1 teaspoon of black pepper

Instructions:

1. Using a bowl, add the shredded leftover turkey breasts and seasonings. Mix it with your washed hands until it mixes properly.
2. Roll out the tortilla wraps thinly and avoid breaking or cracking any tortillas.
3. Using a bowl, add and beat the eggs.
4. Brush the egg wash on both sides and allow it to refrigerate for 30 minutes.
5. After thirty minutes, remove the tortilla wraps and cut it into 8 spring roll sheets.
6. Fill the shredded leftover turkey into each sheet.
7. Roll each turkey into a spring roll and brush it with the egg wash.
8. Place it inside your air fryer and cook it for 5 minutes at a 360 degrees Fahrenheit.

Nutritional Information per serving:

Calories: 45, Fat: 2g, Protein: 5g, Dietary Fiber: 0g,

Carbohydrates: 0.2g

Chapter 5: Air Fryer Dinner Recipes

General Wong's Beef and Broccoli

Time: 25 minutes (plus 30 minutes for marinating)

Yield: 4

Ingredients:

- 1 pound of steak, sliced into strips
- 1 pound of stemmed and chopped into florets broccoli
- 1/3 cup of oyster sauce
- 1/3 cup of sherry
- 1 tablespoon of minced ginger
- 1 tablespoon of minced garlic
- 1 tablespoon of olive oil
- 1 tablespoon of soy sauce
- 1 tablespoon of sesame oil
- 1 teaspoon of cornstarch

Instructions:

1. Using a bowl, add the oyster sauce, sherry, minced ginger, minced garlic, olive oil, soy sauce, sesame oil, cornstarch and stir it until it is properly mixed.
2. Then, add the steak, broccoli, cover it well and allow it to marinate for 30 minutes or overnight.
3. Then preheat your air fryer to 360 degrees Fahrenheit.
4. After marinating, place the marinade steak and broccoli in your air fryer.
5. Cook it for 15 minutes at a 360 degrees Fahrenheit or until it is done.
6. Serve and enjoy along with the white rice!

Nutritional Information per serving:

Calories: 340, Fat: 21g, Protein: 21g, Dietary Fiber: 2.5g, Carbohydrates: 18g

Irresistible Meatloaf

Time: 25 minutes

Yield: 4

Ingredients:

- 1 ½ pound of lean ground beef
- 1 beaten egg
- 1 cup of panko breadcrumbs
- 1/3 cup of steak sauce
- 1 finely chopped onion
- 1 chopped green bell pepper
- ½ cup of chopped mushrooms
- 1 tablespoon of chopped thyme
- 1 teaspoon of paprika
- 1 teaspoon of garlic powder
- 1 teaspoon of salt
- 1 teaspoon of black pepper

Instructions:

1. Preheat your air fryer to 390 degrees Fahrenheit.
2. Using a large bowl, add all the ingredients and stir until it mixes properly.
3. Thereafter, grease a heat-safe pan or the air fryer baking accessory with a nonstick cooking spray.
4. Add the mixed ground beef into the pan or baking accessory and flatten the top.
5. After that, place the pan or accessory inside your air fryer and cook it for 25 minutes at a 390 degrees Fahrenheit or until it gets brown and done.
6. Thereafter, carefully remove it from your air fryer and allow it to cool off before serving.
7. Serve and enjoy!

Nutritional Information per serving:

Calories: 300, Fat: 18g, Protein: 23g, Dietary fiber: 0.7g, Carbohydrates: 9g

Rockstar Rib Eye-Steak

Time: 20 minutes

Yield: 1 or 2

Ingredients:

- 2 pounds of rib-eye steak
- 1 tablespoon of olive oil
- 1 teaspoon of salt
- 1 teaspoon of black pepper
- 1 teaspoon of ground coriander
- 1 teaspoon of brown sugar
- 1 teaspoon of sweet paprika
- 1 teaspoon of mustard powder
- 1 teaspoon of onion powder
- 1 teaspoon of chili powder
- 1 teaspoon of garlic powder

Instructions:

1. Preheat your air fryer to 390 degrees Fahrenheit.
2. Sprinkle the olive oil over the rib-eye steak.
3. Season the steak on all sides with all the listed seasonings until it is well covered.
4. Place the steak into your air fryer basket.
5. Cook it for 8 minutes at a 390 degrees Fahrenheit.
6. After 8 minutes, flip the steak over and cook for an additional 7 minutes.
7. When done, carefully remove the steak from your air fryer and allow it to cool off before serving.
8. Serve and enjoy!

Nutritional Information per serving:

Calories: 520, Fat: 35g, Dietary Fiber: 0g, Carbohydrates: 2g, Protein: 56g

Super-Yummy Roast Pork Belly

Time:

Yield: 2

Ingredients:

- 2 pounds of pork belly
- 2 teaspoons of garlic powder
- 2 teaspoons of onion powder
- 1 teaspoon of smoked paprika
- 1 teaspoon of salt
- 2 teaspoons of five-spice powder
- 2 teaspoons of rosemary
- 1 teaspoon of black pepper

Instructions:

1. Fill a large pot with enough water, boil it and then add the pork belly into the hot water for 10 minutes.
2. Then remove it from the boiling water and allow it to dry for 3 hours or until it dries completely.
3. Use a fork to poke some holes all around the pork belly.
4. While still doing that, using a small mixing bowl, add and mix all the seasonings together, then rub the pork belly with the seasonings.
5. Preheat your air fryer to 320 degrees Fahrenheit.
6. Place the pork belly inside your air fryer and cook it for 30 minutes.
7. Increase the temperature to 360 degrees Fahrenheit and cook it for an additional 20 minutes.
8. Serve and enjoy!

Nutritional Information per serving:

Calories: 240, Fat: 20g, Protein: 13g, Dietary Fiber: 0g, Carbohydrates: 1g

Outstanding Rack of Lamb

Time: 25 minutes

Yield: 4

Ingredients:

- 2 racks of lamb
- ¼ cup of freshly chopped parsley
- 4 cloves of minced garlic
- 2 tablespoons of olive oil
- 2 tablespoons of honey
- 1 teaspoon of salt
- 1 teaspoon of black pepper

Instructions:

1. Preheat your air fryer to 390 degrees Fahrenheit.
2. Using a blender or food processor, add the parsley, garlic cloves, olive oil, honey, salt, and black pepper and blend it until it gets totally grounded.
3. Rub the grounded parsley-garlic on the lamb racks, without using them all as you will need them later.
4. Put the grill pan accessory into your air fryer, and place the lamb racks on top.
5. Cook it for 15 minutes at a 390 degrees Fahrenheit or until it gets brown in color.
6. Spread another layer of the puree on the lamb racks.
7. Serve and enjoy!

Nutritional Information per serving:

Calories: 335, Fat: 26g, Protein: 21g, Dietary Fiber: 0g, Carbohydrates: 2.5g

Phenomenal Herbed Roast Beef

Time: 1 hour

Yield: 4

Ingredients:

- 4-pound roasted beef
- 1 tablespoon of olive oil
- 1 teaspoon of salt
- 1 teaspoon of black pepper
- 1 teaspoon of dried thyme
- 1 tablespoon of freshly chopped rosemary
- 1 tablespoon of freshly chopped parsley

Instructions:

1. Preheat your air fryer to 360 degrees Fahrenheit.
2. Using a bowl, add and mix the olive oil, salt, black pepper, thyme, rosemary, parsley properly.
3. Rub the mixture all over the roasted beef.
4. Place the beef inside your air fryer basket and cook it for 20 minutes.
5. After 20 minutes, flip the beef over and cook for an additional 30 minutes or until it reaches your desired preference.
6. Remove the roasted beef and allow it to cool of before serving.
7. Serve and enjoy!

Nutritional Information per serving:

Calories: 210, Fat: 10g, Protein: 27g, Dietary Fiber: 0.2g, Carbohydrates: 0.6g

Amazing Lamb Chops with Herbed Garlic Sauce

Time: 25 minutes

Yield: 4

Ingredients:

- 4 lamb chops
- 1 garlic bulb
- 1 tablespoon of freshly chopped parsley
- 1 tablespoon of freshly chopped oregano
- 2 tablespoons of olive oil
- 1 teaspoon of onion powder
- 1 teaspoon of salt
- 1 teaspoon of black pepper

Instructions:

1. Preheat your air fryer to 390 degrees Fahrenheit.
2. Brush the garlic bulb with an olive oil and place it inside your air fryer, cook it for 12 minutes or until it is properly roasted, then remove it from your air fryer and set it aside.
3. Using a small bowl, mix the parsley, oregano, olive oil, onion powder, salt, and the black pepper properly.
4. Thereafter spread each lamb chop with about one teaspoon of the herbed olive oil mixture.
5. Place the lamb chops into your air fryer and cook it for 6 minutes at a 390 degrees Fahrenheit or until it turns brown.
6. Press the garlic cloves with a garlic press and mix it properly with the herbed olive oil.
7. Spread the garlic sauce over the lamb chops.
8. Serve and enjoy!

Nutritional Information per serving:

Calories: 180, Fat: 8g, Protein: 23g, Carbohydrates: 1.7g, Dietary Fiber: 0.5g

Chapter 6: Air Fryer Appetizer Recipes

Astonishing Chicken Kebabs

Time: 15 minutes

Yield: 2

Ingredients:

- 2 chopped boneless, skinless chicken breasts
- 6 halves of mushrooms
- 1 chopped red bell pepper
- 1 chopped green bell pepper
- 1 chopped yellow bell pepper
- 1/3 cup of honey
- 1/3 cup of soy sauce
- 1 teaspoon of salt
- 1 teaspoon of black pepper
- Wooden skewers

Instructions:

1. Preheat your air fryer to 340 degrees Fahrenheit.
2. Using a bowl, add and mix 1/3 cup of honey, 1/3 cup of soy sauce, salt, and black pepper.
3. For each wooden skewer, add the bell peppers, chicken, and mushroom slices.
4. Thereafter, brush the chicken kabobs with the honey soy sauce mixture.
5. Place the chicken kabobs into your air fryer basket and cook it for 15 to 20 minutes.
6. Serve and enjoy!

Nutritional Information per serving:

Calories: 90, Fat: 14g, Protein: 8g, Dietary Fiber: 1g, Carbohydrates: 6g

Appetizing Avocado Fries

Time: 20 minutes

Yield: 4

Ingredients:

- 2 avocados, peeled, pitted, and sliced into fries
- 1 cup of panko breadcrumbs
- 1 teaspoon of salt

Instructions:

1. Preheat your air fryer to 390 degrees Fahrenheit.
2. Using a bowl, mix the panko breadcrumbs with 1 teaspoon of salt.
3. Dredge the avocado fries into the panko breadcrumb mixture until it is properly covered.
4. Place the avocado fries inside your air fryer, cook it for 10 minutes and then shake it 5 minutes after that.
5. Serve and enjoy!

Nutritional Information per serving:

Calories: 130, Fat: 11g, Protein: 4g, Dietary Fiber: 4g, Carbohydrates: 6g

Godly Pork Taquitos

Time: 25 minutes

Yield: 4

Ingredients:

- 30-ounces of cooked and shredded pork tenderloin
- 2 ½ cups of shredded mozzarella cheese
- 10 small whole wheat tortillas
- 1 lime juice

Instructions:

1. Preheat your air fryer to 380 degrees Fahrenheit.
2. Stir the lime juice over the shredded pork tenderloins.
3. Soften the tortillas in your air fryer by microwaving it for 10 seconds.
4. For each tortilla add 3-ounces of the shredded pork and ¼ cup of the mozzarella cheese.
5. lightly roll up the tortillas.
6. Then spray a nonstick cooking spray over the tortillas and place it inside your air fryer.
7. Cook it for 7 to 10 minutes or until it gets a golden brown color, and then flip after 5 minutes.
8. Serve and enjoy!

Nutritional Information per serving:

Calories: 210, Fat: 29g, Protein: 7g, Dietary Fiber: 3g, Carbohydrates: 15g

Gratifying Stuffed Mushrooms

Time: 35 minutes

Yield: 2

Ingredients:

- 6 mushrooms
- ½ cup of peeled and chopped onion
- 1 tablespoon of breadcrumbs
- 1 teaspoon of garlic puree
- 1 tablespoon of olive oil
- 1 teaspoon of freshly chopped parsley
- 1 teaspoon of salt
- 1 teaspoon of black pepper

Instructions:

1. Using a bowl, add the onion, breadcrumbs, garlic puree, olive oil, parsley, salt, and black pepper.
2. Remove the middle stalk of each mushroom and fill them with the onion mixture.
3. Grease your air fryer basket and place the stuffed mushrooms into it.
4. Cook it for 10 minutes at a 360 degrees Fahrenheit.
5. Once done, carefully remove it from your air fryer and cook it for 10 minutes.
6. Serve and enjoy!

Nutritional Information per serving:

Calories: 80, Fat; 7g, Protein: 6g, Carbohydrates: 5g, Dietary Fiber: 2.5g

Everyday Chicken Nuggets

Time: 17 minutes

Yield: 2

Ingredients:

- 1 pound of boneless, skinless chicken breasts, cut into 1-inch pieces
- 1 beaten egg
- 1 cup of milk
- 2 cups of flour
- 1 cup of breadcrumbs
- 2 teaspoons of salt
- 1 teaspoon of black pepper
- 1 teaspoon of sweet paprika

Instructions:

1. Preheat your air fryer to 360 degrees Fahrenheit.
2. Using a bowl, mix the eggs and milk properly.
3. Pick a second bowl, add the flour and place it aside.
4. Then using a third bowl, add the breadcrumbs, salt, black pepper, sweet paprika and mix properly.
5. Dredge the chicken pieces in the flour, soak the chicken pieces into the egg wash, and then cover it with the seasoned breadcrumbs.
6. Place the chicken pieces in your air fryer and cook it for 10 minutes at a 360 degrees Fahrenheit or until it has a golden brown color, flipping halfway through.
7. Serve and enjoy!

Nutritional Information per serving:

Calories: 190, Fat: 9g, Protein: 7g, Dietary Fiber: 1g, Carbohydrates: 20g

Chapter 7: Air Fryer Poultry Recipes

Flavorful Fried Chicken

Time: 30 minutes

Yield: 4

Ingredients:

- 4 small chicken thighs
- 1 cup of flour
- 1 cup of breadcrumbs
- 2 beaten eggs
- 1 teaspoon of salt
- 1 tablespoon of Cajun seasoning

Instructions:

1. Preheat your air fryer to 390 degrees Fahrenheit.
2. Using three bowls, add the flour to the first bowl, in the second bowl add the eggs and beat it properly, and in the third bowl add the breadcrumbs, salt, Cajun seasoning and mix properly.
3. Dredge the chicken thighs in the flour, immerse it into the egg mixture, and cover it with the breadcrumbs.
4. Grease your air fryer basket with a nonstick cooking spray and put in the 4 chicken thighs inside.
5. Cook it for 25 minutes until the chicken is crispy and turns golden brown.
6. Serve and enjoy!

Nutritional Information per serving:

Calories: 200, Fat: 22g, Protein: 19g, Dietary Fiber: 0g, Carbohydrates: 19g

Delectable Whole Roast Chicken

Time: 50 minutes

Yield: 4

Ingredients:

- 1 (4-pound) whole chicken
- 1 tablespoon of olive oil
- 1 teaspoon of salt
- 1 teaspoon of black pepper
- 1 teaspoon of paprika
- 1 teaspoon of onion powder
- 1 teaspoon of garlic powder
- 1 teaspoon of Italian seasoning
- 1 teaspoon of brown sugar
- 1 tablespoon of dried thyme
- 1 tablespoon of dried oregano
- 1 tablespoon of cayenne pepper

Instructions:

1. Preheat your air fryer to 340 degrees Fahrenheit.
2. Sprinkle the whole chicken with olive oil and rub the seasoning all over.
3. Grease your air fryer basket with a nonstick cooking spray and add the chicken to it.
4. Cook the chicken inside your air fryer for 30 minutes at a 340 degrees Fahrenheit.
5. After 30 minutes, flip the chicken and cook it for an additional 20 minutes or until it is totally done.
6. Serve and enjoy!

Nutritional Information per serving:

Calories: 155, Fat: 3.8g, Dietary Fiber: 0g, Carbohydrates: 0g, Protein: 28g

Divine Buffalo Wings

Time: 25 minutes (plus 4 hours of marinating time)

Yield: 4

Ingredients:

- 2 pounds of chicken wings
- 3 tablespoons of melted butter
- ¼ cup of hot sauce
- 1 teaspoon of paprika
- 1 teaspoon of cayenne pepper
- 1 teaspoon of salt
- 1 teaspoon of black pepper

Buffalo Sauce Ingredients:

- 3 tablespoons of melted butter
- ¼ cup of hot sauce

Instructions:

1. Using a separate bowl, add 3 tablespoons of melted butter, ¼ cup of hot sauce, paprika, cayenne pepper, salt, black pepper, chicken wings and allow it to marinate for 4 hours or overnight.
2. Preheat your air fryer to 390 degrees Fahrenheit.
3. Lubricate your air fryer basket with a nonstick cooking spray and add half of the chicken wings.
4. Cook the chicken wings for 14 minutes, then shake it 7 minutes after and repeat this with the other batch.
5. Using another bowl, add 3 tablespoons of melted butter and ¼ cup of hot sauce.
6. Remove the chicken wings from your air fryer and combine it with the buffalo sauce.
7. Serve and enjoy!

Nutritional Information per serving:

Calories: 240, Fat: 15.5g, Protein: 8g, Carbohydrates: 5g, Dietary Fiber: 6g

Flavorsome Honey Lime Chicken Wings

Time: 30 minutes

Yield: 4

Ingredients:

- 2 pounds of chicken wings
- ¼ cup of honey
- 2 tablespoons of lime juice
- 1 tablespoon of lime
- 1 pressed clove of garlic
- 1 teaspoon of salt
- 1 teaspoon of black pepper

Instructions:

1. Preheat your air fryer to 360 degrees Fahrenheit.
2. Using a bowl, mix the honey, lime juice, lime zest, garlic clove, salt, and black pepper.
3. Add the chicken wings and toss it until it is well covered with the honey-lime mixture.
4. Working in batches, add half of the chicken wings into the air fryer.
5. Cook it for 25 to 30 minutes or until it turns golden brown and crispy, while shaking it every 8 minutes.
6. Serve and enjoy!

Nutritional Information per serving:

Calories: 280, Fat: 25g, Dietary Fiber: 0.2g, Carbohydrates: 3.6g, Protein: 23g

Delightful Coconut Crusted Chicken Tenders

Time: 30 minutes

Yield: 4

Ingredients:

- 1 pound of chicken tender
- 3 beaten eggs
- 2 cups of sweetened shredded coconut
- 1 cup of cornstarch
- 1 teaspoon of salt
- 1 teaspoon of black pepper
- 1 teaspoon of cayenne pepper

Instructions:

1. Preheat your air fryer to 360 degrees Fahrenheit.
2. Using three bowls, add the cornstarch, salt, black pepper, and cayenne pepper into the first bowl. Then in the second bowl, add the eggs and beat it until it mixes properly. While in the third bowl, add the shredded coconut.
3. Dredge each chicken tender in the cornstarch mixture, then dip it into the egg wash, and then cover it with the shredded coconut.
4. Grease your air fryer with a non-stick cooking spray and add the chicken tenders.
5. Cook for 8 minutes at a 360 degrees Fahrenheit or until it turns golden brown.
6. Serve and enjoy!

Nutritional Information per serving:

Calories: 345, Fat: 11g, Protein: 32g, Carbohydrates: 9g, Dietary Fiber: 2.4g

Well-Tasted Popcorn Chicken

Time: 20 minutes

Yield: 2

Ingredients:

- 2 boneless, skinless chicken breasts
- 1 cup of breadcrumbs
- 2 beaten eggs
- 1 cup of flour
- 1 teaspoon of salt
- 1 teaspoon of black pepper
- 1 teaspoon of onion powder
- 1 teaspoon of garlic powder

Instructions:

1. Preheat your air fryer to 390 degrees Fahrenheit.
2. Using a food processor, add the chicken breasts and beat it until it minced properly.
3. Using two bowls, add the flour ,the eggs and mix it properly into the first bowl, then in the second bowl, add the breadcrumbs, seasonings and mix it properly.
4. Mold the minced chicken into small balls.
5. Cover the minced chicken in the flour, dip it into the egg wash, and then cover it with the seasoned breadcrumbs.
6. Place it inside your air fryer and cook it for 10 minutes at a 390 degrees Fahrenheit or until it is fully done.
7. Serve and enjoy!

Nutritional Information per serving:

Calories: 170, Fat: 17g, Protein: 14g, Dietary fiber: 0g, Carbohydrates: 13g

Easy Chicken Strips

Time: 20 minutes

Yield: 2

Ingredients:

- 2 boneless, skinless chicken breasts, sliced into strips
- ½ cup of shredded coconut
- ½ cup of oats
- 1 cup of panko breadcrumbs
- 1 cup of flour
- 2 beaten eggs
- 1 teaspoon of salt
- 1 teaspoon of black pepper
- 1 teaspoon of onion powder
- ½ teaspoon of garlic powder
- 1 teaspoon of smoked paprika

Instructions:

1. Preheat your air fryer to 360 degrees Fahrenheit.
2. Firstly, slice the chicken breasts into thin strips.
3. Using a bowl, add the oats, shredded coconut, breadcrumbs, seasonings and mix properly.
4. Pick a second bowl, add the egg and mix properly, then pick another bowl, add the flour and place it aside.
5. Dredge the strips in the flour, dip the strips into the egg wash, and cover it with the coconut breadcrumb mixture.
6. Grease your air fryer basket with a nonstick cooking spray.
7. Place the chicken breasts inside your air fryer and cook it for 8 minutes at a 360 degrees Fahrenheit.
8. Reduce the heat to 340 degrees Fahrenheit and cook it for an additional 5 minutes until it is done.
9. Serve and enjoy!

Nutritional Information per serving:

Calories: 130, Fat: 12g, Protein: 14g, Carbohydrates: 8g, Dietary Fiber: 0.9g

Savory Sriracha Chicken Drumsticks

Time: 1 hour

Yield: 6

Ingredients:

- 6 drumsticks
- 1 cup of sriracha
- ½ cup of honey
- ½ cup of melted butter
- 1 tablespoon of soy sauce
- 4 cloves of minced garlic
- 1 teaspoon of salt
- 1 teaspoon of black pepper

Instructions:

1. Preheat your air fryer to 390 degrees Fahrenheit.
2. Grease your air fryer basket with a nonstick cooking spray and add the chicken drumsticks.
3. Cook it inside your air fryer for 10 minutes at a 390 degrees Fahrenheit.
4. While still doing that, using a small bowl, add and mix the remaining ingredients.
5. After 10 minutes, remove the chicken drumsticks and brush it with the sriracha sauce.
6. Lower the heat to 360 degrees Fahrenheit and cook the drumsticks for an additional 10 minutes.
7. With the remaining sauce, microwave it inside your air fryer for 30 seconds or at most 1 minute.
8. Carefully remove the chicken drumsticks from your air fryer and cover it with the sriracha sauce again.
9. Serve and enjoy!

Nutritional Information per serving:

Calories: 290, Fat: 36g, Protein: 13g, Dietary Fiber: 0g, Carbohydrates: 22g

Chinese-Style Honey Garlic Chicken

Time: 35 minutes (plus 4 hours of marinating time)

Yield: 4

Ingredients:

- 1 pound of chicken wings
- 1 tablespoon of olive oil
- ¼ cup of soy sauce
- 3 cloves of minced garlic
- 1/3 cup of honey
- 1 teaspoon of white vinegar
- 1 teaspoon of garlic salt
- Green onions (for garnishing purpose)
- Sesame seeds (for garnishing purpose)

Instructions:

1. Using a bowl, add and mix the olive oil, soy sauce, garlic cloves, honey, white vinegar, and the garlic salt properly.
2. Add the chicken breasts and toss it until it gets properly covered.
3. Using a Ziploc bag, add the chicken wings, honey-garlic mixture and allow it to marinate for 4 hours or overnight.
4. Preheat your air fryer to 390 degrees Fahrenheit.
5. Using your baking accessory, add the chicken wings and honey-garlic mixture.
6. Place it inside your air fryer and cook it for 8 minutes at a 390 degrees Fahrenheit.
7. After 8 minutes, stir the chicken wings inside your baking accessory and cook it for an additional 10 minutes, then increase the temperature to 400 degrees Fahrenheit.
8. Garnish it with the green onions and the sesame seeds.
9. Serve and enjoy!

Nutritional Information per serving:

Calories: 200, Fat: 25g, Dietary Fiber: 0.1g, Carbohydrates: 8g, Protein: 27g

Rich Parmesan Crusted Chicken Breasts

Time: 30 minutes

Yield: 4

Ingredients:

- 4 small boneless, skinless chicken breasts
- 1 cup of panko bread crumbs
- ½ cup of Parmesan cheese
- 3 tablespoons of freshly chopped parsley
- 1 teaspoon of salt
- 1 teaspoon of black pepper
- 3 tablespoons of melted butter
- 3 tablespoons of fresh lime juice
- 2 garlic pressed cloves

Instructions:

1. Preheat your air fryer to 360 degrees Fahrenheit.
2. Using a bowl, add and mix the panko breadcrumbs, Parmesan cheese, parsley, salt, and the black pepper properly.
3. Pick another bowl, and mix the melted butter, fresh lime juice, and garlic.
4. Soak the chicken breasts into the butter mixture and cover it with the panko breadcrumb mixture until it is properly covered.
5. Grease your air fryer basket with a nonstick cooking spray and place the chicken breasts inside.
6. Cook it for 20 to 25 minutes inside your air fryer under a 360 degrees Fahrenheit of heat or until it turns golden brown and has a crispy texture.
7. Serve and enjoy!

Nutritional Information per serving:

Calories: 290, Fat: 16g, Protein: 59g, Dietary Fiber: 0.5g, Carbohydrates: 2.6g

Nashville Flaming Hot Breaded Chicken

Time: 35 minutes

Yield: 4

Ingredients:

- 4 medium or small chicken thighs
- 1 cup of buttermilk
- 2 beaten eggs
- ¼ cup of hot sauce

Flour Ingredients:

- 2 cups of flour
- 1 tablespoon of baking powder
- 1 tablespoon of cayenne pepper

Seasoning Spiced Rub Ingredients:

- 2 teaspoons of salt
- 2 teaspoons of paprika
- 2 teaspoons of onion powder
- 2 teaspoons of garlic powder
- 2 teaspoons of chili powder
- 2 teaspoons of black pepper
- 2 teaspoons of dried oregano
- 2 teaspoons of dried basil
- 1 tablespoon of cayenne pepper

Hot Sauce Ingredients:

- 2 tablespoons of hot sauce
- 2 tablespoons of melted butter
- 1 tablespoon of cayenne pepper
- 1 tablespoon of brown sugar
- 1 teaspoon of smoked paprika
- ¾ cup of olive oil

Instructions:

1. Using a small bowl, add and mix all the seasoning spiced rub ingredients properly.
2. Rub the chicken thighs with the seasoning mix and reserve any leftovers.
3. For the battered chicken: using a bowl, add and mix the buttermilk, eggs, and the ¼ cup of hot sauce properly.
4. Using another bowl, add 2 cups of flour, 1 tablespoon of baking powder, 1 tablespoon of cayenne pepper, any leftover spice rub and stir until it is properly mixed.
5. Dredge each chicken thigh into the flour, dip it into the buttermilk mixture and cover it with the flour once again.
6. Preheat your air fryer to 360 degrees Fahrenheit.
7. Place the chicken thighs into your air fryer and cook it for 8 minutes or until its done.
8. Thereafter, carefully remove it from your air fryer and allow it to cool off.
9. Using a small bowl, add and mix all the hot sauce ingredients, pour over the cooked chicken thighs and toss it until it is properly covered.
10. Serve and enjoy!

Nutritional Information per serving:

Calories: 380, Fat: 28g, Protein: 55g, Dietary Fiber: 3.5g, Carbohydrates: 19g

Desirable Korean Fried Chicken Wings

Time: 20 minutes

Yield: 4

Ingredients:

- 1 pound of chicken wings
- ½ cup of cornstarch
- 1 teaspoon of salt
- 1 teaspoon of black pepper
- 1 tablespoon of sesame seeds (for garnishing purposes)

Korean Dressing Ingredients:

- 4 tablespoons of Korean gojuchang
- 1 tablespoon of apple cider vinegar
- 1 tablespoon of melted butter
- 2 tablespoons of honey
- 1 tablespoon of soy sauce

Instructions:

1. Preheat your air fryer to 360 degrees Fahrenheit.
2. Using a bowl, season the chicken wings with the salt and black pepper.
3. Cover the chicken wings with the cornstarch.
4. Grease your air fryer basket with a nonstick cooking spray and add the chicken wings.
5. Cook it for 25 to 30 minutes or until it gets crispy, while still shaking it at a regular intervals of 8 minutes.
6. Using a bowl, add and mix all the Korean dressing ingredients properly.
7. Thereafter, carefully remove it from your air fryer and toss it with the Korean dressing mixture.
8. Garnish it with the sesame seeds.
9. Serve and enjoy!

Nutritional Information per serving:

Calories: 260, Fat: 16g, Protein: 15g, Dietary Fiber: 0.5g, Carbohydrates: 12g

Awesome Crispy Baked Garlic Parmesan Chicken Wings

Time: 40 minutes

Yield: 2

Ingredients:

- 1 pound of chicken wings
- 1 tablespoon of olive oil
- 2 tablespoons of melted butter
- 4 cloves of minced garlic
- 3 tablespoons of freshly chopped parsley
- 1 teaspoon of salt
- ½ cup of grated Parmesan cheese

Instructions:

1. Using a large pot, fill it with water and place a steamer basket into it.
2. Add the chicken wings on top of the steamer basket and allow it to steam for 12 minutes. Once it is done, remove it from the steamer basket and let it get cool off and dry.
3. Preheat your air fryer to 390 degrees Fahrenheit.
4. Grease your air fryer basket with a nonstick cooking spray and add the chicken wings.
5. Cook the chicken wings for 25 to 30 minutes or until it has a golden brown color and a crispy texture, while still shaking it at a regular intervals of 8minutes.
6. Using a saucepan, mix properly the olive oil, melted butter, garlic cloves, parsley, and the salt, while heating it on an average pressure of heat for 3 minutes. Thereafter remove and place it aside.
7. Remove the chicken wings from your air fryer and place it into a large bowl, pour the garlic mixture over the chicken wings and toss until it is properly covered.
8. Sprinkle the Parmesan cheese on it.
9. Serve and enjoy!

Nutritional Information per serving:

Calories: 510, Fat: 40g, Protein: 35g, Dietary Fiber: 0g, Carbohydrates: 3g

Spicy Teriyaki Chicken Wings

Time: 30 minutes (plus 4 hours of marinating time)

Yield: 4

Ingredients:

- 1 ½ pound of chicken wings
- ½ cup of soy sauce
- ¼ cup of rice wine vinegar
- ¼ cup of brown sugar
- 3 cloves of minced garlic
- 1 teaspoon of ginger powder
- 1 teaspoon of red pepper flakes
- 1 teaspoon of salt
- 1 teaspoon of black pepper

Instructions:

1. Using a bowl, add and mix the soy sauce, rice wine vinegar, brown sugar, garlic cloves, ginger powder, red pepper flakes, salt, and black pepper.
2. Then using a Ziploc bag, add the chicken wings, teriyaki mixture and allow it to marinate for 4 hours or overnight.
3. Preheat your air fryer to 390 degrees Fahrenheit.
4. Using your baking accessory, add the chicken wings and marinade it.
5. Place it inside your air fryer and cook it for 8 minutes at a pressure of 390 degrees Fahrenheit.
6. After 8 minutes, flip the chicken over and cook it for an additional 10 minutes, at this point increasing the temperature to 400 degrees Fahrenheit.
7. Serve and enjoy!

Nutritional Information per serving:

Calories: 220, Fat: 15g, Protein: 17g, Dietary Fiber: 0g, Carbohydrates: 3g

Chapter 8: Air Fryer Fish and Seafood

Remarkable Fish and Chips with Sauce

Time: 35 minutes

Yield: 4

Fish Ingredients:

- 4 cod fish fillets
- 1 teaspoon of olive oil
- 1 cup of flour
- 1 cup of panko breadcrumbs
- 2 beaten eggs

Fries Ingredients:

- 2 potatoes, cut into ½-inch strips
- 1 tablespoon of olive oil
- 1 teaspoon of salt

Sauce Ingredients:

- ¼ cup of mayonnaise
- 1 tablespoon of freshly chopped dill
- 1 tablespoon of freshly chopped tarragon
- 2 tablespoons of sour cream
- 2 tablespoons of finely chopped dill pickle
- 2 tablespoons of finely chopped red onion

Instructions:

1. Soak the potato pieces in a bowl of water for 30 minutes. After 30 minutes, drain it into a colander and pat it dry using a cloth.
2. Preheat your air fryer to 360 degrees Fahrenheit.
3. Using a large bowl, add and mix the potato strips, olive oil, salt and toss it until it is properly covered.
4. Place the potato strips inside your air fryer and cook it for 20 to 25 minutes, while still shaking it at a regular interval of 6 minutes until the potatoes

reaches its golden brown color and crispy texture state. After that, remove and set it aside.

5. Then for the fish: Using a bowl, add the flour, pick another bowl, add the eggs and stir properly, then using another separate bowl, add the breadcrumbs and olive oil.
6. Dredge the cod fillets in the flour, dip it in the egg mixture, and then cover it with the breadcrumbs.
7. Grease your air fryer basket with a nonstick cooking spray and add the battered cod fillets.
8. Cook it for 10 minutes or until it has a golden brown color, carefully remove it from your air fryer basket and allow it to cool off.
9. For the sauce: Using a bowl, add all the mayonnaise, dill, tarragon, sour cream, dill pickle, the red onion, and stir it until it is properly mixed .
10. Serve and enjoy!

Nutritional Information per serving:

Calories: 250, Fat: 8g, Protein: 13g, Dietary Fiber: 2g, Carbohydrates: 3g

Grand Air-Fried Coconut Shrimp

Time:

Yield: 4

Ingredients:

- 1 pound of peeled and deveined shrimp
- 1 cup of shredded coconut
- 1 cup of panko breadcrumbs
- 2 eggs
- 1/3 cup of flour
- 1 teaspoon of salt
- 1 teaspoon of black pepper

Instructions:

1. Preheat your air fryer to 360 degrees Fahrenheit.
2. Using a bowl, add and mix the flour, salt, and black pepper. Then using a second bowl, add the eggs and beat it properly. Pick a third bowl, add and mix the shredded coconut and breadcrumbs.
3. Dredge each shrimp in the flour, dip it into the egg wash and then cover it with the coconut breadcrumb mixture.
4. Grease your air fryer basket with a nonstick cooking spray and add the shrimp.
5. Cook it for 10 to 15 minutes at a 360 degrees Fahrenheit or until it has a golden brown color.
6. Serve and enjoy!

'Nutritional Information per serving:

Calories: 250, Fat: 14g, Protein: 9g, Dietary Fiber: 1.6g, Carbohydrates: 4g

Splendid Salmon Patties

Time: 15 minutes

Yield: 2

Ingredients:

- 1 (14-ounce) can of drained canned salmon
- ¼ cup of chopped onion
- ¼ cup of ground oats
- ¼ cup of wheat flour
- 1 egg
- ¼ cup of mayonnaise
- 1 tablespoon of parsley
- 1 teaspoon of salt
- 1 teaspoon of black pepper
- 1 cup of breadcrumbs

Instructions:

1. Preheat your air fryer to 390 degrees Fahrenheit.
2. Using a bowl, add and mix the canned salmon, onion, ground oats, wheat flour, egg, parsley, salt, black pepper and the mayonnaise properly.
3. Divide the salmon mixture into 4 patties and cover it with the breadcrumbs.
4. Add the salmon patties inside your air fryer and cook it for 8 to 10 minutes or until it has a golden brown color.
5. Serve and enjoy!

Nutritional Information per serving:

Calories: 260, Fat: 15g, Protein: 16g, Dietary Fiber: 1g, Carbohydrates: 14g

Japanese-Style Fried Prawns

Time: 15 minutes

Yield: 2

Ingredients:

- 1 pound of peeled and deveined prawns
- 1 cup of rice flour
- 1 cup of panko bread crumbs
- 2 eggs
- 1 teaspoon of ground ginger
- 1 tablespoon of paprika
- 1 teaspoon of salt
- 1 teaspoon of black pepper
- 1 teaspoon of garlic powder

Instructions:

1. Preheat your air fryer to 380 degrees Fahrenheit.
2. Using a bowl, add the prawns, salt, black pepper, garlic powder, ground ginger and toss until it is properly mixed.
3. Then using another bowl, add the rice flour, paprika and mix it well. Pick a second bowl, add the eggs and beat it properly. Then using a third bowl, add the panko breadcrumbs.
4. Dredge the seasoned prawns into the flour, dip it into the egg wash, and then cover it with the panko breadcrumbs.
5. Grease your air fryer basket with a nonstick cooking spray and add the prawns.
6. Cook it for 8 minutes or until it has a golden brown color and repeat if necessary.
7. Serve and enjoy!

Nutritional Information per serving:

Calories: 210, Fat: 8g, Protein: 40g, Dietary Fiber: 0g, Carbohydrates: 4g

Great Air-Fried Soft-Shell Crab

Time:

Yield: 2

Ingredients:

- 2 soft-shell crabs
- 1 cup of flour
- 2 beaten eggs
- 1 cup of panko breadcrumbs
- 1 teaspoon of onion powder
- 1 teaspoon of garlic powder
- 1 teaspoon of salt
- 1 teaspoon of black pepper

Instructions:

1. Preheat your air fryer to 360 degrees Fahrenheit.
2. Using a bowl, add the flour, pick a second bowl, add the eggs and mix properly. Then using a third bowl, mix the panko breadcrumbs and the seasonings properly.
3. Grease your air fryer basket with a nonstick cooking spray and add the crabs inside.
4. Cook it inside your air fryer for 8 minutes or until it has a golden brown color.
5. Thereafter, carefully remove it from your air fryer and allow it to cool off.
6. Serve and enjoy!

Nutritional Information per serving:

Calories: 380, Fat: 16g, Protein: 24g, Carbohydrates: 9g, Dietary Fiber: 5g

Stunning Air-Fried Clams

Time: 15 minutes

Yield: 2

Ingredients:

- 1 (10-ounce) can of whole baby clams, drained and shucked
- 2 beaten eggs
- 1 cup of flour
- 1 cup of panko breadcrumbs
- 1 teaspoon of salt
- 1 teaspoon of black pepper
- 1 teaspoon of garlic powder
- 1 teaspoon of onion powder
- 1 teaspoon of cayenne pepper
- 1 tablespoon of dried oregano

Instructions:

1. Preheat your air fryer to 390 degrees Fahrenheit.
2. Using a bowl, add the flour, pick a second bowl, add the eggs and mix properly. Then using a third bowl, add and mix the panko breadcrumbs, seasonings, and the herbs properly.
3. Dredge the clams in the flour, immerse it into the egg wash and then cover it with the breadcrumb mixture.
4. Place the clams inside your air fryer and cook it for 2 minutes or until it has a golden brown color, while being cautious of overcooking.
5. Thereafter, carefully remove it from your air fryer and allow it to cool.
6. Serve and enjoy!

Nutritional Information per serving:

Calories: 225, Fat: 12g, Protein: 15g, Carbohydrates: 3g, Dietary Fiber: 0.5g

Mind-Blowing Air-Fried Crawfish with Cajun Dipping Sauce

Time: 10 minutes

Yield: 4

Ingredients:

- 1 pound of cooked craw-fish tail meat
- 1 beaten egg
- 4 chopped green onions
- 1 teaspoon of melted butter
- 1 teaspoon of salt
- 1 teaspoon of cayenne pepper
- 1 teaspoon of black pepper
- 1/3 cup of panko breadcrumbs
- 1/3 cup of bread flour

Sauce Ingredients:

- ¾ cup of mayonnaise
- ½ cup of ketchup
- 1 teaspoon of horseradish

Instructions:

1. Preheat your air fryer to 380 degrees Fahrenheit.
2. Using a bowl, add the eggs, green onion, butter, salt, cayenne pepper, black pepper and salt.
3. Add the panko breadcrumbs, bread flour and pour in the craw-fish, stirring it until it is properly covered.
4. Grease your air fryer basket with a nonstick cooking spray.
5. Add the battered craw-fish inside your air fryer and cook it for 5 minutes or until it has a golden brown color.
6. Thereafter, using a bowl, add the mayonnaise, ketchup, horseradish and mix properly.
7. Serve and enjoy!

Nutritional Information per serving:

Calories: 205, Fat: 16.7g, Protein: 26g, Dietary Fiber: 0.3g, Carbohydrates: 8.8g

Southern-Air-Fried Cat Fish

Time: 15 minutes

Yield: 4

Ingredients:

- 4 skinless catfish fillets
- 1 teaspoon of salt
- 1 teaspoon of black pepper
- 1 cup of cornmeal
- 1 cup of flour

Instructions:

1. Preheat your air fryer to 360 degrees Fahrenheit.
2. Using a bowl, add the cornmeal, flour, salt, black pepper and mix it properly.
3. Dredge the catfish fillets in the seasoned cornmeal mixture.
4. Grease your air fryer with a non-stick cooking spray and add the catfish fillets.
5. Cook the catfish for 8 minutes at a 360 degrees Fahrenheit or until it turns brown.
6. Serve and enjoy!

Nutritional Information per serving:

Calories: 350, Fat: 15g, Protein: 25g, Dietary Fiber: 0g, Carbohydrates: 36g

Wondrous Creole Fried Shrimp with Sriracha Sauce

Time: 10 minutes

Yield: 4

Ingredients:

- 1 pound of peeled and deveined shrimp
- ½ cup of cornmeal
- ½ cup of breadcrumbs
- 1 beaten egg
- 1 tablespoon of hot sauce
- 1 tablespoon of mustard
- 2 tablespoons of creole seasoning
- 1 teaspoon of onion powder
- 1 teaspoon of garlic powder
- 1 teaspoon of black pepper
- 1 teaspoon of salt

Siracha Sauce Ingredients:

- 1 cup of mayonnaise
- 3 tablespoons of sriracha sauce
- 1 tablespoon of soy sauce
- 1 teaspoon of black pepper

Instructions:

1. Preheat your air fryer to 360 degrees Fahrenheit.
2. Using a bowl, add the eggs, hot sauce, mustard, 1 tablespoon of creole seasoning, onion powder, garlic powder, black pepper, salt, the shrimp and toss until it is properly covered.
3. Using another bowl, add the breadcrumbs, flour, 1 tablespoon of creole seasoning, the shrimp and cover it properly.
4. Grease your air fryer basket with a nonstick cooking spray and add the shrimp.
5. Cook for it for 5 minutes or until it has a golden brown color, while being careful not to overcook.
6. Thereafter, carefully remove it from your air fryer and allow it to cool.

7. Pick a separate bowl, add and mix all the sauce ingredients properly.
8. Serve!

Nutritional Information per serving:

Calories: 200, Fat: 12g, Protein: 15g, Carbohydrates: 7g, Dietary Fiber: 0.6g

Chapter 9: Air Fryer Meat Recipes

Sweet and Spicy Montreal Steak

Time: 15 minutes

Yield: 2

Ingredients:

- 2 boneless sirloin steaks
- 1 tablespoon of olive oil
- 1 tablespoon of brown sugar
- 1 tablespoon of Montreal steak seasoning
- 1 teaspoon of crushed red pepper

Instructions:

1. Preheat your air fryer to 390 degrees Fahrenheit.
2. Sprinkle the sirloin steaks with olive oil.
3. Rub each steak with the brown sugar, Montreal steak seasoning, and the crushed red pepper.
4. Place the baking accessory inside your air fryer and add it to the steaks inside.
5. Cook it for 3 minutes at a 390 degrees Fahrenheit.
6. After 3 minutes has elapsed, flip the steak over and cook it for an additional 3 minutes or until it reaches your desired texture.
7. Carefully remove it from your air fryer and allow it to cool before slicing them into strips.
8. Serve and enjoy!

Nutritional Information per serving:

Calories: 160, Fat: 5g, Protein: 25g, Dietary Fiber: 0g, Carbohydrates: 3g

Stunning Chicken Sandwich

Time: 25 minutes

Yield: 2

Ingredients:

- 2 boneless, skinless chicken breasts
- 1 cup of flour
- 2 beaten eggs
- 1 teaspoon of garlic powder
- 1 teaspoon of onion powder
- 1 teaspoon of salt
- 1 teaspoon of black pepper
- 4 toasted hamburger buns

Instructions:

1. Using a bowl, add and mix the flour and seasonings properly. Then in a second bowl, add the eggs and beat it well.
2. Dip the chicken breasts into the egg mixture and remove any excess batter.
3. Dredge the chicken breasts in the flour mixture until it is properly coated.
4. Preheat your air fryer to 340 degrees Fahrenheit.
5. Grease your air fryer basket with a nonstick cooking spray.
6. Add the chicken breasts and cook for 6 minutes at a 340 degrees Fahrenheit.
7. Flip the chicken breasts and cook it for an additional 6 minutes.
8. Then increase the temperature to 400 degrees Fahrenheit and cook it for 2 minutes per side.
9. Serve and enjoy on the toasted hamburger buns, or with any toppings you desire!

Nutritional Information per serving:

Calories: 265, Fat:1 7g, Protein: 21g, Dietary Fiber: 1.2g, Carbohydrates: 5g

Hearty Hot Dogs

Time: 10 minutes

Yield: 2

Ingredients:

- 2 hot dogs
- 2 hot dog buns
- Any hot dog toppings if desired

Instructions:

1. Preheat your air fryer to 390 degrees Fahrenheit.
2. Put the hot dogs inside your air fryer and cook it for 5 minutes.
3. Carefully remove it from your air fryer and allow it to cool off.
4. Place the cooked hot dogs in the bun and add any desired toppings.
5. Serve and enjoy!

Nutritional Information per serving:

Calories: 110, Fat: 10g, Protein: 5g, Dietary Fiber: 0g, Carbohydrates: 2g

Sweet and Sour Pork

Time: 30 minutes

Yield: 4

Ingredients:

- 2 pounds of chopped into 1-inch pieces boneless pork
- 2 beaten eggs
- 1 cup of cornstarch
- 3 tablespoons of oil
- 1 teaspoon of salt
- 1 teaspoon of black pepper

Sweet and Sour Sauce Ingredients:

- ½ cup of sugar
- 5 tablespoons of ketchup
- ½ cup of seasoned rice vinegar
- 1 tablespoon of soy sauce
- ½ teaspoon of salt

Instructions:

1. Preheat your air fryer to 340 degrees Fahrenheit.
2. Using a bowl, add the eggs and beat it properly. Pick another bowl, add and mix the cornstarch, salt, black pepper and properly and set it aside.
3. Dredge each pork chunks into the cornstarch mixture, dip it in the egg wash, and then cover it with the cornstarch mixture.
4. Grease your air fryer basket with a nonstick cooking spray.
5. Place the pork chunks in your air fryer basket and cook it for 8 to 12 minutes at a 340 degrees Fahrenheit, shaking it halfway through.
6. Then, using a saucepan, add all the sweet and sour sauce ingredients and heat it under an average pressure of heat for around 5 minutes, while still stirring consistently.
7. Once the pork turns golden brown and crispy, carefully remove it from your air fryer and allow it to cool off.
8. Serve and enjoy with the sauce!

Nutritional Information per serving:

Calories: 360, Fat: 19g, Protein: 14g, Dietary Fiber: 0g, Carbohydrates: 6g

Yummy Rodeo Sirloin Steaks with Coffee Rub

Time: 25 minutes

Yield: 2

Ingredients:

- 2 boneless sirloin steaks
- 1 tablespoon of olive oil
- 2 tablespoons of ground coffee
- 1 tablespoon of salt
- 1 tablespoon of brown sugar
- 1 tablespoon of dried thyme
- 1 teaspoon of garlic powder
- 1 teaspoon of black pepper

Instructions:

1. Preheat your air fryer to 390 degrees Fahrenheit.
2. Sprinkle the sirloin steak with the olive oil.
3. Using a bowl, add the ground coffee, salt, brown sugar, dried thyme, garlic powder, black pepper and mix properly.
4. Rub each sirloin steak with the coffee rub until it is properly covered.
5. Place the baking accessory inside your air fryer and add it to the steak inside.
6. Cook it for 3 minutes at a 390 degrees Fahrenheit.
7. After 3 minutes, flip the steak over and cook for an additional 3 minutes or until it reaches your desired texture.
8. Carefully remove it from your air fryer and allow it to cool before slicing.
9. Serve and enjoy!

Nutritional Information per serving:

Calories: 480, Fat: 29g, Protein: 45g, Carbohydrates: 8g, Dietary Fiber: 0.2g

Chapter 10: Air Fryer Vegetable and Sides Recipes

Supreme Air-Fried Tofu

Time: 55 minutes

Yield: 4

Ingredients:

- 1 block of pressed and sliced into 1-inch cubes of extra-firm tofu
- 2 tablespoons of soy sauce
- 1 teaspoon of seasoned rice vinegar
- 2 teaspoons of toasted sesame oil
- 1 tablespoon of cornstarch

Instructions:

1. Using a bowl, add and toss the tofu, soy sauce, seasoned rice vinegar, sesame oil until it is properly covered.
2. Place it inside your refrigerator and allow to marinate for 30 minutes.
3. Preheat your air fryer to 370 degrees Fahrenheit.
4. Add the cornstarch to the tofu mixture and toss it until it is properly covered.
5. Grease your air fryer basket with a nonstick cooking spray and add the tofu inside your basket.
6. Cook it for 20 minutes at a 370 degrees Fahrenheit, and shake it after 10 minutes.
7. Serve and enjoy!

Nutritional Information per serving:

Calories: 80, Fat: 5.8g, Protein: 5g, Carbohydrates: 3g, Dietary Fiber: 1.2g

Not Your Average Zucchini Parmesan Chips

Time: 15 minutes

Yield: 4

Ingredients:

- 2 thinly sliced zucchinis
- 1 beaten egg
- ½ cup of panko breadcrumbs
- ½ cup of grated Parmesan cheese
- 1 teaspoon of salt
- 1 teaspoon of black pepper

Instructions:

1. Prepare your zucchini by using a mandolin or a knife to slice the zucchinis thinly.
2. Use a cloth to pat dry the zucchini chips.
3. Then using a bowl, add the eggs and beat it properly. After that, pick another bowl, and add the breadcrumbs, Parmesan cheese, salt, and black pepper.
4. Dredge the zucchini chips into the egg mixture and then cover it with the Parmesan-breadcrumb mixture.
5. Grease the battered zucchini chips with a nonstick cooking spray and place it inside your air fryer.
6. Cook it for 8 minutes at a 350 degrees Fahrenheit.
7. Once done, carefully remove it from your air fryer and sprinkle another teaspoon of salt to give it some taste.
8. Serve and enjoy!

Nutritional Information per serving:

Calories: 100, Fat: 16g, Protein: 4g, Carbohydrates 9g, Dietary Fiber: 1.8g

Outstanding Batter-Fried Scallions

Time: 10 minutes

Yield: 4

Ingredients:

- 4 bunches of trimmed scallions
- 1 cup of flour
- 1 cup of white wine
- 1 teaspoon of salt
- 1 teaspoon of black pepper

Instructions:

1. Preheat your air fryer to 390 degrees Fahrenheit.
2. Using a bowl, add and mix the white wine, the flour and stir until it gets smooth.
3. Add the salt, the black pepper and mix again.
4. Dip each scallion into the flour mixture until it is properly covered and remove any excess batter.
5. Grease your air fryer basket with a nonstick cooking spray and add the scallions. At this point, you may need to work in batches.
6. Cook the scallions for 3 to 5 minutes or until it has a golden brown color and crispy texture, while still shaking it after every 2 minutes.
7. Carefully remove it from your air fryer and check if it's properly done. Then allow it to cool before serving.
8. Serve and enjoy!

Nutritional Information per serving:

Calories: 190, Fat: 22g, Protein: 4g, Carbohydrates: 9g, Dietary Fiber: 0.8g

Delectable French Green Beans with Shallots and Almonds

Time: 25 minutes

Yield: 4

Ingredients:

- 1 ½ pounds of stemmed French green beans
- ½ pound of peeled, stemmed quartered shallots
- ¼ cup of lightly toasted silvered almonds
- 2 tablespoons of olive oil
- 1 tablespoon of salt
- 1 teaspoon of garlic salt
- 1 teaspoon of white pepper

Instructions:

1. Using a large pot, fill it with water and boil it under an average pressure of heat.
2. Add the green beans, a tablespoon of salt, stir for a while and cook it for 2 minutes.
3. Once done, drain it using a colander and allow it to cool off.
4. Using a large bowl, add the green beans, shallots, garlic salt, white pepper, olive oil and toss it until it is properly covered.
5. Place the green beans and shallots inside your air fryer basket and cook it for 25 minutes at a 400 degrees Fahrenheit, shaking it halfway through.
6. Then pick a large bowl, add the cooked green beans, shallots, almonds and toss it until it is properly covered.
7. Serve and enjoy!

Nutritional Information per serving:

Calories: 110, Fat: 9g, Protein: 3g, Carbohydrates: 7g, Dietary Fiber: 4g

Super-Healthy Air-Fried Green Tomatoes

Time: 25 minutes

Yield: 4

Ingredients:

- 4 sliced into ¼-inch pieces green tomatoes
- 2 beaten eggs
- 2 tablespoons of milk
- 1 cup of flour
- ½ cup of cornmeal
- ½ cup of panko breadcrumbs
- 1 teaspoon of garlic powder
- 1 teaspoon of paprika
- 1 teaspoon of salt
- 1 teaspoon of black pepper

Instructions:

1. Using a bowl, add 1 cup of flour.
2. Pick a second bowl, add the eggs, milk and mix properly.
3. Using a third bowl, add the cornmeal, panko breadcrumbs, seasonings and mix properly.
4. For each tomato slice, dredge it in the flour, dip it into the egg mixture and then cover it with the cornmeal-breadcrumb mixture.
5. Grease your air fryer basket with a nonstick cooking spray.
6. Working in batches, add the green tomatoes, cook it for 20 minutes at a 360 degrees Fahrenheit of heat, and flip it after 10 minutes.
7. Repeat the above step with any leftover.
8. Serve and enjoy!

Nutritional Information per serving:

Calories: 190, Fat: 12g, Protein: 4g, Dietary Fiber: 6g, Protein: 4.25g

Luscious Air-Fried Broccoli Crisps

Time: 35 minutes

Yield: 4

Ingredients:

- 1 large chopped into florets broccoli head
- 2 tablespoons of olive oil
- 1 teaspoon of salt
- 1 teaspoon of black pepper

Instructions:

1. Preheat your air fryer to 360 degrees Fahrenheit.
2. Using a bowl, add and toss the broccoli florets with the olive oil, salt, and black pepper.
3. Add the broccoli florets and cook it for 12 minutes, then shake after 6 minutes.
4. Carefully remove it from your air fryer and allow it to cool off.
5. Serve and enjoy!

Nutritional Information per serving:

Calories: 120, Fat: 19g, Protein: 4.5g, Carbohydrates: 8.3g, Dietary Fiber: 4.5g

Chapter 11: Air Fryer Desert Recipes

Toothsome Caramel Cheesecake

Time: 1 hour

Yield: 8

Crust Ingredients

- 2 cups of graham cracker crumbs
- ¼ cup of brown sugar
- ½ cup of melted butter

Filling Ingredients:

- 3 (8-ounce) package of softened cream cheese
- 1 cup of brown sugar
- 3 eggs
- ¾ cup of whipping cream
- ¼ cup of coffee syrup

Caramel Sauce Ingredients:

- ½ cup of butter
- 1 ¼ cup of brown sugar
- 2 tablespoons of coffee syrup
- ½ cup of whipping cream
- 1 teaspoon of salt

Instructions:

1. Preheat your air fryer to 360 degrees Fahrenheit.
2. Apply the flour to the sides and bottoms of a spring form pan.
3. Using a bowl, add and mix all the crust ingredients properly.
4. Press the crust down into the spring form pan.
5. Then using a large mixing bowl, add and beat all the filling ingredients properly.
6. Pour the filling over the crust.
7. Place it inside your air fryer and cook it for 15 minutes.

8. Reduce the heat to 320 degrees Fahrenheit and cook it for 10 more minutes.
9. Finally, reduce the heat to 300 degrees Fahrenheit and cook it for 15 minutes.
10. Then, carefully remove it from the oven and refrigerate it for 6 hours or overnight.
11. Thereafter, using a saucepan, melt the butter under an average pressure of heat.
12. Add the brown sugar, salt, coffee syrup and mix them properly.
13. Boil and cook it for 1 minute, while still stirring consistently until the brown sugar liquefies.
14. Pour in the whipping cream, turn off the heat and thereafter allow it to cool off for 10 minutes.
15. Spread the caramel sauce over the cheesecake.
16. Serve and enjoy!

Nutritional Information per serving:

Calories: 420, Fat: 25g, Protein: 5g, Dietary Fiber: 0g, Carbohydrates: 10g

Conclusion

Hopefully, after going through this book and trying out a couple of recipes, you will get to understand the flexibility and utility of the air fryers. It is certainly a multipurpose kitchen appliance that is highly recommended to everybody as it presents one with a palatable atmosphere to enjoy fried foods that are not only delicious but healthy, cheaper, and more convenient. The use of this kitchen appliance ensures that the making of some of your favorite snacks and meals will be carried out in a stress free manner without hassling around, which invariably legitimizes its worth and gives you a value for your money.

This book will be your all-time guide to understanding the basics of the air fryer and Ketogenic Diet, because with all the recipes mentioned in the book, it is rest assured that it will be something that you and the rest of the people around the world will enjoy for the rest of your lives. Also after going through this book , you will be able to prepare delicious and flavorsome meals that will not only be easy to carry out, but tasty and healthy as well.

However, you should never limit yourself to the recipes solely mentioned in this cookbook, go on and try new things! Explore new recipes! Experiment with different ingredients, seasonings and different methods! Create some new recipes and keep your mind open. By so doing you will be able to get the best out of your air fryer.

In a nutshell, if you found this book helpful, please kindly take the time to leave an honest review on Amazon. Your feedback will be greatly appreciated. Thank you, and the best wishes to you!